Peter Dabrock, Mat
Jens Ried (F

Individualized Medicine
between Hype and Hope

Individualized Medicine between Hype and Hope

Exploring Ethical and Societal Challenges for Healthcare

edited by

Peter Dabrock, Matthias Braun, Jens Ried

LIT

This publication is part of a research project funded by the
federal ministry of education and research (01GP1186)

Gedruckt auf alterungsbeständigem Werkdruckpapier entsprechend
ANSI Z3948   DIN ISO 9706

Bibliographic information published by the Deutsche Nationalbibliothek
The Deutsche Nationalbibliothek lists this publication in the Deutsche
Nationalbibliografie; detailed bibliographic data are available in the Internet at
http://dnb.d-nb.de.

ISBN 978-3-643-90298-6

A catalogue record for this book is available from the British Library

©LIT VERLAG GmbH & Co. KG Wien,
Zweigniederlassung Zürich 2012
Klosbachstr. 107
CH-8032 Zürich
Tel. +41 (0) 44-251 75 05
Fax +41 (0) 44-251 75 06
e-Mail: zuerich@lit-verlag.ch
http://www.lit-verlag.ch

LIT VERLAG Dr. W. Hopf
Berlin 2012
Fresnostr. 2
D-48159 Münster
Tel. +49 (0) 2 51-620 320
Fax +49 (0) 2 51-23 19 72
e-Mail: lit@lit-verlag.de
http://www.lit-verlag.de

Distribution:
In Germany: LIT Verlag Fresnostr. 2, D-48159 Münster
Tel. +49 (0) 2 51-620 32 22, Fax +49 (0) 2 51-922 60 99, e-mail: vertrieb@lit-verlag.de

In Austria: Medienlogistik Pichler-ÖBZ, e-mail: mlo@medien-logistik.at
In Switzerland: B + M Buch- und Medienvertrieb, e-mail: order@buch-medien.ch
In the UK: Global Book Marketing, e-mail: mo@centralbooks.com
In North America: International Specialized Book Services, e-mail: orders@isbs.com

Content

i

Content

Individualized Medicine between Hype and Hope

Under the catchphrase of "Individualized Medicine"[1] efforts are currently being made – besides other definitions and expectations[2] – to get to the matter of chances and risks of a biomarker-based medicine and healthcare system. The promise of this change in medicine and healthcare – often also described with the adjectives "personalized" or "customized" – lies in wanting to develop more precise diagnoses on the one hand and therapies better customized to the individual affected and possible preventions on the other hand,[3] partly by combining information on diseases, ways of life and environmental conditions with a biomarker analysis, especially on the molecular level[4]. It is and will remain controversial whether costs are lowered by such a biomarker-based differentiation of medical regimes ("health economy efficiency")[5] or whether costs are increased by gaining and progressing information additionally needed[6]. In any case, what is intended is the

---

[1] A. M. Laberge, W. Burke, "Personalized Medicine and Genomics", in: The Hastings Center (Ed.), *From Birth to Death and Bench to Clinic: The Hastings Center Bioethics Briefing Book for Journalists, Policymakers, and Campaigns*, NY 2008, p. 133-136; A. M. Laberge, W. Burke, "Clinical and public health implications of emerging genetic technologies", in: *Seminars in Nephrology*, 30(2)/2010, p. 185-194.

[2] B. Hüsing, J. Hartig, B. Bührlen, T. Reiß, S. Gaisser (Eds.), *Individualisierte Medizin und Gesundheitssystem*, TAB-Arbeitsbericht 126, Berlin 2008.

[3] See Department of Health and Human Services (HHS) (Eds.), *Health, United States, 2007,* Washington DC 2007; M. Dion-Labrie, M.-C. Fortin, M.-J. Hébert, H. Doucet, "The use of Personalized Medicine for patient selection for renal transplantation: Physicians' views on the clinical and ethical implications", *BMC Medical Ethics*, 11(5)/2010.

[4] See V. Ozdemir, D. Husereau, S. Hyland, S. Samper, M. Z. Salleh, "Personalized Medicine Beyond Genomics: New Technologies, Global Health Diplomacy and Anticipatory Governance", in: *Current Pharmacogenomics and Personalized Medicine*, 7(4)/2009, p. 225-230.

[5] See Personalized Medicine Coalition, "The case for Personalized Medicine"; http://www.personalizedmedicinecoalition.org/sites/default/files/files/Case_for_PM_3rd_edition.pdf.

[6] See B. Hüsing et al., *Individualisierte Medizin und Gesundheitssystem*.

1

increase of preventive, diagnostic and therapeutic efficiency ("medical efficiency") by avoiding overmedication, too little or incorrect medication with "blockbuster"-applications as well as by the precision of the doses needed. Individualized, Personalized or Customized Medicine symbolizes the vision of a medicine in the (post-)genomic age, in which "-omics"-knowledge is to be used for the benefits of medicine and healthcare.[7]

Besides such hopes and partly pretentious expectations of a more precise medicine with less side effects and possibly even lower costs for the healthcare system,[8] the vision of the so-called Individualized Medicine meets with scepticism and concerns.[9] Such sceptical or even adverse reactions refer to the probability of a realization of the propagated visions and/or the social consequences predicted. On the one hand it is thus to be doubted whether the promises can really be fulfilled: The so-called Individualized Medicine is rather considered a new hype of biotechnology that has to be demythologized and whose reasons and interests have to be uncovered.[10] On the other hand, even though the prospect of the development

---

[7] See M. Gadebusch Bondio, S. Michl, "Die neue Medizin und ihre Versprechen", in: *Deutsches Ärzteblatt*, 107(21)/2010, A-1062, B-934, C-922.

[8] See HHS, *Health, United States*; Personalized Medicine Coalition, "The case for Personalized Medicine"; H. Bolouri (Ed.), *Personal Genomics and Personalized Medicine*, London 2010, B. Obama, *President's Council of Advisors on Science and Technology. Priorities for Personalized Medicine*; http://www.ostp.gov/galleries/PCAST/pcast_report_v2.pdf, A. Merkel, *Rede von Bundeskanzlerin Angela Merkel beim Zukunftskongress Gesundheitswirtschaft des Bundesgesundheitsministeriums*; http://www.bundesregierung.de/Content/DE/Rede/2010/04/2010-04-29-merkel-zukunftskongress.html, A. Schavan, *Ideen – Innovation – Wachstum. Hightech-Strategie 2020 für Deutschland*; http://www.bmbf.de/pub/hts_2020.pdf.

[9] See N. Rose, "Race, risk and medicine in the age of ‚your own personal genome'", in: *BioSocieties*, 3/2008, p. 423-439; R. Kollek, T. Lemke, *Der medizinische Blick in die Zukunft. Gesellschaftliche Implikationen prädiktiver Gentests*, Frankfurt a. M./NY 2008; R. Kollek, Gesellschaftliche Aspekte der "Individualisierten Medizin". Beitrag zum "Expertengespräch mit Diskussion des TAB-Zukunftsreports: Individualisierte Medizin und Gesundheitssystem"; http://www.hf-initiative.de/fileadmin/dokumente/ProGesundheit_9_2009.pdf; N. W. Paul, "Die Medizin nimmt's persönlich. Möglichkeiten und Grenzen der Individualisierung von Diagnose und Therapie, Vortrag im Forum Bioethik des Deutschen Ethikrates am 24. Juni 2009"; http://www.ethikrat.org/dateien/pdf/FB_2009-06-24_Praesentation_Paul.pdf; M. J. Khoury, J. Evans, W. Burke, "A reality check for personalized medicine", in: *Nature*, 464(7289)/2010, p. 680.

[10] K. Peterson-Iyer, "Pharmacogenomics, Ethics, and Public Policy", in: *Kennedy Institute of Ethics Journal*, 18(1)/2008, p. 35-56.

of (more) customized medication is not seen as utopian, the social consequences are regarded as rather or even extremely harmful: The concept of a
"person of genetic risk" would undermine the traditional concept of social
solidarity in the healthcare system and would therefore lead to a govern-
mentalization of one's own life that is hidden behind the euphemistic label
of "autonomy" and that is often not explicitly known.[11] Since it could not be
counted on the condition that these medical high technologies will be covered by healthcare systems founded on solidarity or owned by the state, the
increase of inequality in healthcare has to be taken into account.[12] Furthermore the increase of costs in the healthcare market could not be excluded.
What would have to be feared are further negative effects on the doctor-
patient-relationship or subtle social alterations when dealing with personal
data ("privacy") or even the re-emergence of categories which were deemed
to be overcome such as the category of "race".[13]

While there are already numerous studies, researches and essays that –
often according to their interests which are not always disclosed – give a
one-sided portrayal of either the advantages or the disadvantages of the
accordingly staged vision of the so-called Individualized Medicine, the
ELSI-questions relevant and urging in this field are considered occasionally, however, up to now they are mostly not analysed in a systematic way.
Thus the assessment of the so-called Individualized Medicine formed of
different disciplines, joined through dialogue and resulting in an interdisciplinary and governmentally transdisciplinary perspective, as well as, above
all, its existing evaluations ("the observation of the observers"[14]) is a research desideratum; this collection of essays aims at contributing to the
elimination of this desideratum.

The range of topics of the Individualized Medicine as well as of its
existing critique or advocacy staged in the media and in economy proves

---

[11] T. Lemke, "Die Genetifizierung der Medizin. Dimensionen, Entwicklungsdynamiken und Folgen", in: *Widerspruch*, 29(56)/2009, p. 49-65.

[12] See B. Prainsack, "Die Verflüssigung der Norm – Selbstregierung und personalisierte Gesundheit", in: B. Paul, H. Schmidt-Semisch (Eds.), *Risiko Gesundheit. Über Risiken und Nebenwirkungen der Gesundheitsgesellschaft*, Wiesbaden 2010.

[13] See N. Rose, "Race, risk and medicine"; T. Ingold, "When biology goes underground: genes and the spectre of race", in: *Genomics, Society and Policy*, 3(2)/2009, p. 23-37.

[14] N. Luhmann, *Soziale Systeme: Grundriss einer allgemeinen Theorie*. Edited by Suhrkamp [2006], Frankfurt a. M. 1984.

to be of special importance for such considerations of the second or third order, particularly because it inhabits a nearly unique, highly ambivalent intermediate position between hope and hype compared to other biomedical visions of the future: Though there have been only few medical and healthcare-economical results in the so-called Individualized Medicine so far; such breakthroughs are vainly expected in other biotechnological or medical visions of the future, e.g. in stem cell research, genetic therapy or in parts of synthetic biology. These successes – especially in the field of pharmacogenomics – are definitely presentable, such as genetic pretests that allow a so far unknown precision of medication with epilepsy, carzinoma or cardiovascular diseases.[15] However, with the help of these successes, the whole vision up to an almost utopian scenario of a medicine based on molecules customized to the individual is promoted as realistic (and thus worth funding) – and this is the other side of the assessment of the so-called Individualized Medicine. The whole bunch of yet unsolved technical and regulatory problems, which would have to be dealt with in order to at least widen the present state of development sustainably, fades away in the light of the mentioned rash conclusion drawn between the few successes and a utopian vision. The fact that the promoters do not publicly face the yet mostly unsolved issues of technology and governance of genetic testing, of biobank regimes or public-health-genomic strategies and as a consequence thereof the health-information-technology-complex suf-

---

[15] S. Paik, G. Tang, S. Shak, C. Kim, J. Baker, W. Kim, M. Cronin, F. L. Baehner, D. Watson, J. Bryant, J. P. Costantino, C. E. Geyer, D. L. Wickerham, N. Wolmark, "Gene expression and benefit of chemotherapy in women with node-negative, estrogen receptor–positive breast cancer", in: *Journal of Clinical Oncology*, 24(23)/2006, p. 3726-3734; C. W. Tate, A. D. Robertson, R. Zolty, S. F. Shakar, J. Lindenfeld, E. E. Wolfel, M. R. Bristow, B. D. Lowes, "Quality of life and prognosis in heart failure: results of the Beta-Blocker Evaluation of Survival Trial (BEST)", in: *Journal of Cardiac Failure*, 13(9)/2007, p. 732-737; J. Li, A. E. G. Lenferink, Y. Deng, C. Collins, C. Qinghua, E. O. Purisima, M. D. O'Connor-McCourt, E. Wang, "Identification of high-quality cancer prognostic markers and metastasis network modules", in: *Nature Communications*, 1/2010, p. 1-8; D. K. Pal, A. W. Pong, W. K. Chung, "Genetic evaluation and counseling for epilepsy", in: *Nature Reviews Neurology*, 6(8)/2007, p. 445-453; A. Nakagomi, Y. Seino, Y. Endoh, Y. Kusama, H. Atarashi, K. Mizuno, "Upregulation of Monocyte Proinflammatory Cytokine Production by C-Reactive Protein is Significantly Related to Ongoing Myocardial Damage and Future Cardiac Events in Patients With Chronic Heart Failure", in: *Journal of Cardiac Failure*, 16(7)/2010, p. 562-571.

ficiently, but rather avoid them generously when realizing the vision of the Individualized Medicine, increases the necessity to analyse the staging of the so-called Individualized Medicine on the ELSI-levels of a second and third observation.

The contributions collected in this anthology, thematically gathered in three parts, exactly pursue this challenge to discriminate between hope and hype, between realistic and utopian visions and their respective optimistic and pessimistic functionalization and thus also the challenge to ask for the respective consequences and feedback for the ELSI-discourse.

The first part of the collection at hand – *Mapping the Field of Individualized Medicine* – maps out the field of the so-called Individualized Medicine by firstly questioning the plausibility of the assumptions forming the basis of the respective visions and then examining those regarding their relation to the classic terms of medical ethics as well as their historical placement.

Peter Dabrock opens the search for an adequate and evaluating vision assessment of the so-called Individualized Medicine with his fundamental contribution "The Constructed Reality of the So-Called Individualized Medicine – Socio-Ethical and Theological Comments". After firstly deconstructing the challenges and characteristics of the expression 'Individualized Medicine', pleading for a more appropriate use of the term 'stratifying medicine' and a critical discussion of the generally sceptical and critical positions of the so-called Individualized Medicine, the contribution focuses on the ethical and social questions emerging. Apart from the topical ethical and legal questions, the essay expands its focus to the questions newly dealt with due to the biomarker-based medicine of the respectively underlying social self-conceptions and the questions of repercussions and interactions of the so-called 'Individualized Medicine' on the respective understanding of the guiding social principles of 'autonomy', 'solidarity', 'justice', 'community', 'standardization', and 'normality'.

Taking up this question, Diana Aurenque asks for the consequences of the so-called Individualized Medicine regarding the patient's autonomy in her contribution "Personalized Medicine as Encouragement and Discouragement of Patient Autonomy". In doing so, she follows the thesis that the so-called Individualized Medicine can be understood as encouraging and strengthening the patient autonomy on the one hand. This is true when it is mostly aimed at increasing the efficiency and exactness of therapies made (prospectively) possible by Individualized Medicine and potentially preventive models. On the other hand, the essay shows that accompanying (more and more) complexity in medicine and linked to the usage of new and (possibly) further reaching biomarker-based methods, the consequence of such further confidence in the so-called Individualized Medicine could possibly weaken patient autonomy. Due to this ambiguity and the development of the so-called Individualized Medicine that can presently not be foreseen, she develops a set of criteria for the further dealing with the ELSI-questions in the field of the so-called Individualized Medicine.

In his essay "Personalized Healthcare: Focus on Individuality" Harald Matern examines the meaning and consequences of the expressions 'individualized' or even 'personalized' in the concept of a so-called Individualized or Personalized Medicine. While doing so, he assumes that presently there is a discrepancy between the expectations of the patients evoked by the terms 'individualized' and 'personalized' on the one hand and the present state of technical possibilities on the other hand. In order to eliminate and prevent such a one-sided disappointment of expectations, it is essential to look at the respectively fundamental branches of the philosophical and theological debates on the terms of individuality and personality more closely. Such a perspective pursues a double goal: On the one hand it forms a heuristic concept for the further discussion of the relationship between society and economy regarding the communication of new medical – or more generally biotechnological – developments and, accompanying them, the respective self-concept of the modern individual. On the other hand, such a perspective allows the development of a meta-ethical perspective and it allows asking up to which degree the respective philosophical and theological identity concepts can be relevant for an ethical assessment of the so-called Individualized Medicine.

Concluding the first part of this collection, the essay of Reinhard Heil "Stratified Medicine: The Upholding of Eugenic Ideals? Eugenics and Genetic Counseling" examines the question in how far conceptual and structural parallels as well as historical relations can be drawn between a stratifying medicine and eugenics. By presenting and discussing prominent eugenic positions (Francis Galton, Charles Davenport), it is shown that the idea of eugenics is not dependent on certain scientific and political theories, but grows in the most differing social climates, and which challenges thus emerge for the debate on a stratifying medicine.

By evaluating the chances and risks of the so-called Individualized Medicine in the second part of this volume – *Individualized Medicine: Empirical Data* – the focus is set on the question of empirical evidence of the assumed consequences especially regarding the doctor-patient-relationship; this is meant in the sense of concrete ethics as an approach as exact as possible to the topic field in order to ask for particularly normative and in this context especially for the ethical and social aspects of the descriptions building on these descriptive results in the third part of this collection – *Conceptual and Ethical Aspects*. Too little would have been done if the respective empirical contributions – marking the transition between description and normative questioning – did not create connection points for the ELSI-discourse at the same time.

In their essay "Patients' Self-determination in 'Personalized Medicine': The Case of Whole Genome Sequencing and Tissue Banking in Oncology" Tanja Kohnen, Jan Schildmann and Jochen Vollmann ask in how far the patients' self-determination is newly challenged by the Individualized Medicine. In doing so, they examine which new challenges arise for the practice of the 'informed consent' and which necessities are genuine for its theoretical modelling. The contribution develops the model of a 'dynamic-dialogical-consent' as adaptation to the challenges of the so-called Individualized Medicine.

With his contribution "'Everything Better Than 50% Is Better Than Now': An Ethical-Empirical Study of Physicians' and Researchers' Understanding of Individualized Medicine", Arndt Hessling goes one step further in the search for determining concrete challenges by implementing the so-called Individualized Medicine in the clinical practice. His social-empirical study in the context of colorectal carcinoma diseases shows three essential benchmarks for dealing with the so-called Individualized Medicine. Firstly, there is the question of dealing with the proneness to errors of biomarker-based tests; secondly, there is the question for possible changes in the doctor-patient-relationship; and thirdly, there is the question of dealing with and storing the data that is very delicate for the most part.

Introducing the third part of this volume – *Conceptual and Ethical Aspects* – Arndt Bialobrzeski asks for the intrinsic and extrinsic requirements for implementing a biomarker-based medicine into the healthcare system in his essay "On the Value of Privacy in Individualized Medicine". As one of the essential thresholds he identifies the integration of biobanks on an organizational level as well as into the scientific research structure and taking that up, the development of privacy regimes that are considered as safe and trustworthy by society. On a theoretical level, the essay analyses different conceptions of privacy in order to thus develop a framework model for the further dealing with biobanks as a prerequisite for the development of the so-called Individualized Medicine.

The question whether the different dealings with privacy or perhaps even a new social understanding of 'privacy' leads to a new culture of autonomy, is dealt with by Martin Langanke, Tobias Fischer and Kyle Brothers in their contribution "Public Health – It Is Running through My Veins: Personalized Medicine and Individual Responsibility for Health". In doing so, they illustrate that the assumed connection between the so-called Individualized Medicine and autonomy is far less obvious than the debates on the individual's healthcare have assumed so far.

Reflecting the observations of the Individualized Medicine itself and thus giving a further perspective on the question of an observing reflection of the observation as asked at the beginning, Konrad Ott and Tobias Fischer deal with the critical objections against the so-called Individualized Medicine in their essay "Can Objections to Individualized Medicine be Justified?" by applying Foucault's term of bio-politics such as the 'cura sui'. Thus, they follow the hypothesis that the term 'cura sui' does not have to be opposed to the idea of a biomarker-based medicine, but that the discussion of the ideas behind it can essentially contribute to a healthcare system that takes into account the challenges of the modern age.

In their essay "Individualized Medicine: Ethical and Social Challenges" Matthias Braun and Jens Ried take up the considerations on the prerequisites of the so-called Individualized Medicine as well as the determination of the relation of the challenges of Individualized Medicine and autonomy by focussing their discussion once again on concrete ethical, legal and social challenges in the field of biomarker-based medicine. By discussing the concept of the person of genetic risk and the present assessments and considerations of the legal state of the so-called Individualized Medicine, the essay votes for a genuine placing of the discourse on biomarker-based medicine in the context of public health research. In this sense, the ELSI-questions in the field of the so-called Individualized Medicine can be dealt with by using the previous methods and tools of medical and bio-ethical research so that the requirements for an attentively accompanying ethical assessment of the chances and risks of the so-called Individualized Medicine are given from an ethical perspective.

The contributions of this collection are based on a conference week pertaining to the topic "Individualisierte Medizin zwischen Hype und Hope. Ethische, rechtliche und soziale Herausforderungen einer in Szene gesetzten Vision" ("Individualized Medicine between Hype and Hope: Ethical, Legal and Social Challenges of a Staged Vision") sponsored by the *Bundesministerium für Bildung und Forschung* (BMBF). The conference was held by the editors at the department of theology in cooperation with the institute of history and medical ethics at the Friedrich-Alexander-University Erlangen-Nuremberg in September/October of 2011. The contributions are the speeches held by the participants of the conference and the invited experts. They were adapted to the results of the discussions during the conference and eventually taken a mutual look at.

Special thanks go to the *Bundesministerium für Bildung und Forschung* for funding the project as well as to the *Deutsches Zentrum für Luft- und Raumfahrt* for the constructive cooperation in carrying out the project. Such a project would not have been possible without the numerous contributors whose commitment and élan helped developing this volume (in alphabetical order): Daniela Appee, Franziska Hofmann, Theresa Lauterbach, Katharina Müller and Johanna Schell. We thank Mr. Bellmann of the *LIT Verlag* for the pleasant and successful cooperation and the excellent care.

Erlangen, May 2012   Peter Dabrock
                                                                     Matthias Braun
                                                                        Jens Ried

The Constructed Reality of the So-Called Individualized Medicine – Socio-Ethical and Theological Comments[1]

Peter DABROCK

1 "If men define situations as real, ... "

"... they are real in their consequences."[2] This sentence, known as Thomas theorem in social studies, could be the heading of the social and thus socio-ethical and theological challenges which the so-called Individualized Medicine entails. No one can tell what exactly Individualized Medicine is. Nevertheless, it is advertised as an existing or soon to be expected medical progress suggesting that the consequences of such claims and expectations will become real. It is the aim of the following deliberations to survey the consequences of linguistic policies but also of social implications including theological interpretations.

In detail: The voluminous assessment report of the study group of the ISI institute in Karlsruhe, headed by Bärbel Hüsing, does not dispense with a heuristic definition[3], but at the same time there is no hope for this proposed definition to be broadly received and accepted. And thus, more than

---

[1] Translated and revised version of the article: "Die konstruierte Realität der sog. individualisierten Medizin – sozialethische und theologische Anmerkungen", in: V. Schumpelick, B. Vogel (Eds.), *Medizin nach Maß: Individualisierte Medizin – Wunsch und Wirklichkeit*, Freiburg 2011, p. 285-313.

[2] "Wenn die Menschen Situationen als real definieren, so sind auch ihre Folgen real." (W. I. Thomas (Ed.), *Person und Sozialverhalten*, Soziologische Texte 26, Neuwied/Berlin 1965, p. 114).

[3] See B. Hüsing, J. Hartig, B. Bührlen, T. Reiß, S. Gaisser (Eds.), *Individualisierte Medizin und Gesundheitssystem*, TAB-Arbeitsbericht 126, Berlin 2008. Here, provisionally, Individualized Medicine is functionally defined as "eine mögliche künftige Gesundheitsversorgung [...], die aus dem synergistischen Zusammenwirken der drei Treiber 'Medizinischer und gesellschaftlicher Bedarf', 'Wissenschaftlich-technische Entwicklungen in den Lebenswissenschaften' und 'Patientenorientierung' entstehen könnte." (B. Hüsing et al., *Individualisierte Medizin und Gesundheitssystem*, p. 7).

only a few use the chance of the still diffuse semantics in order to actively pursue politics of notion or following the Thomas theorem: in order to influence the real consequences of the still open definition of the situation according to their own ways. For one thing, it is obvious: Even though it is still not clear what the term 'Individualized Medicine' exactly means, it sounds compelling. Who could be against a medicine that promises individualization or personalization or customization – naming alternatively coined words that are used equally and of which none has yet replaced another? Quite the opposite: Such a medicine is wanted by almost everyone and almost everyone is willing to invest a lot, especially if this life is understood as the last chance – in allusion to a promising book title.[4]

Thus, the fight for the prerogative of interpretation has already begun. On that point, here are three deconstructively[5] meant observations: firstly, regarding it under a naïve perspective, one could assume that the neologism is an unintentional pleonasm. Since – following this rather naïve wishful thinking – individual reference, accuracy of fit and personality are characteristics of any type of good medicine. Why would a specifying epithet be necessary, which only by its addition creates the impression that no longer all medicine would refer to the individual and be as customized as possible? Even though – having a broad idea of the matter – one knows that Individualized Medicine does mean something else than the medical idea of the ideal physician, who is characterized by sensitivity regarding the suffering patient in his individuality[6]. It has to be stated: Solely the fact that the term 'Individualized Medicine' does not at once cause puzzlement, because only few think it is a pleonasm, must be understood as a phenomenon of crisis

---

[4] See M. Gronemeyer (Ed.), *Das Leben als letzte Gelegenheit: Sicherheitsbedürfnisse und Zeitknappheit,* [2]Darmstadt 1996. Differing from platonic or Far Eastern myths of reincarnation, according to Christian resurrection belief it is the life on earth that is the last chance; however, Christians may believe in the infinite and vital affirmation of life with God; see 1 Cor 15.

[5] According to my understanding, deconstruction does not mean arbitrariness of interpretation or even destruction of sense but an interpretation of texts or other means of communication that pay attention to the background, the unconscious or the screened-off and are sensitive to difference. The consequence is a new production of meaning by differing reconstruction.

[6] See for this idea: K. K. Dörner (Ed.), *Der gute Arzt: Lehrbuch der ärztlichen Grundhaltung,* Schriftenreihe der Akademie für Integrierte Medizin, [2]Stuttgart/NY 2003.

for medicine and the profession of doctors: The current state of medicine or the medical service does no longer evoke the impression that the patient as person or individual is the main priority.

Apart from this first discovery of symptoms of crisis, it has secondly to be asked to what individualization, personalization or customization it refers. Here, too, knowing the matter superficially, one knows that the creative introduction of notions – despite all differences in detail of particular interpretations – mainly refers to differentiations in diagnosis and therapy of diseases that are based on biomarkers.[7] Taking this background seriously, two consequences can be drawn: The reference to the individual either *can* or *should* primarily be built by the scientifically refined medicine, however, not by the so-called talking medicine which has repeatedly been demanded for, but is notoriously underpaid. This insight into linguistic policy developments is thought provoking: This second questioning of the current linguistic policies on this term does not mean that one is against a medicine which is as precise and comes with as little side effects as possible. However, occupying the term 'personality' (even more than the term 'individuality') for a scientific method of differentiation cannot be deemed innocent. Since personality only develops within social togetherness – at least according to the trinity-theological, personalized, phenomenological and socio-psychological traditions[8]. Personality and communication with the other are mutually conditioned. According to this coined interpretation in Europe's philosophical and theological tradition, especially the notion 'personalized medicine' has to be understood as infelicitously chosen if it

---

[7] See B. Hüsing et al., *Individualisierte Medizin und Gesundheitssystem*, p. 8: "Im Kontext der individualisierten Medizin wird insbesondere an die Genom- und Postgenomforschung, die molekulare medizinische Forschung und die zellbiologische Forschung die Erwartung gerichtet, eine Wissens- und Technologiebasis bereitzustellen, von der aus verbesserte Diagnose-, Therapie- und Präventionsmöglichkeiten entwickelt werden können." (See also: B. Hüsing et al., *Individualisierte Medizin und Gesundheitssystem*, p. 71-106) I agree with this axiom of the understanding of the so-called Individualized Medicine and will build the following argumentation on it.

[8] In the English-speaking tradition the notion of 'person' has very different connotations: the main focus lies on conscience and possession. Though these connotations become more and more important, the mentioned connotations oriented at dialog remain plausible, they have to be made a stronger part of the public consciousness again; see J. Heinrichs, K. Stock, Art. "Person", in: TRE, Vol. 26, Berlin/ Boston 1996, p. 220-231.

13

does not imply a medicine oriented towards dialog but a medicine relying on refined biomedical processes.

Thirdly, in view of linguistic policies regarding the term 'Individualized Medicine' one has to consider: When, for the reasons given, preferring the notions 'individualized' or 'customized' medicine to the notion of 'Personalized' Medicine because of stating the importance on a bioscience level of individual biomarkers that are supposed to specify given therapy options and to avoid wrong therapies, however, without claiming to substitute the social dimension important for personality, then, nevertheless, the experts will quickly state: We are far away from achieving a really *individualized* medicine in the sense of an exactly fitting medicine for each and every patient. This assessment is based on biomedical and economical reasons.[9] On a biomedical level the sequencing and mapping of the human genome has opened up the access to molecular medicine; but the more time has passed, the more it has become obvious how extremely complex the cross-linking is within the genome and between the genome, the intra-organismic environment, which is analyzed by other -omics-sciences, the extra-organismic environment that the organism is exposed to, and the behavior and eating habits of each individual. Achieving an exactly fitting individualization of diagnostics and therapy in this interaction is extremely difficult, extremely time-consuming and extremely expensive – and this is the second skeptical objection – and thus it becomes almost impossible in the near future. After all, it would not only be the individual genome that had to be sequenced, which is – despite dropping costs – still too expensive, but also other biomarkers would constantly have to be checked and observed in order to be able to note the differences over the pass of time. In any case it is hardly imaginable how such truly individualized approaches could be established in a public health care system. Promising a real individualization is too boastful and can only disappoint, especially when focusing on biomarker-based therapy.

By explaining these three observations against the (too) promising term 'Individualized Medicine' in a deconstructive way, it is not implied that it is

---

[9]   See the work of B. Hüsing et al., *Individualisierte Medizin und Gesundheitssystem*, and as an overview M. Gadebusch Bondio, S. Michl,"Individualisierte Medizin. Die neue Medizin und ihre Versprechen.", in: *Deutsches Ärzteblatt*, 107(21)/2010, p. A-1062, B-934, C-922.

per se a faulty approach to develop a kind of medicine that wants to newly focus on biomarker analysis. However, there are two conclusions that can be drawn from the language criticism outlined: Either one takes advantage of a too grandiose vision with consequences according to the Thomas theorem mentioned at the beginning (which often means disadvantages for other developments) or one disassociates oneself from a promise whose fulfillment is not yet in sight but without giving up on the idea of an exactly fitting medicine with better therapeutic effects and less side effects. Opting for the second consequence on the level of language, it could be preferable to use more modest, but yet more realistic alternatives like the possible terms of stratified or stratifying medicine instead of the critically viewed terms. The use of the term *'Stratified Medicine'* shows that what remains is the big goal of the so-called Individualized Medicine to develop exactly fitting diagnosis and therapy based on biomarkers, but what is dispensed with are too grandiose promises.

The marketing and strategy departments of pharmaceutical companies or others that expect profits from introducing the label 'Individualized Medicine' may believe that attention and money can only be gained by hyping. However, there are many results from trust research that support the assumption that sustainable trust can be created for rather complex goals especially by not raising too high expectations and not making unfulfillable promises which will lead to disappointment and frustration as can be expected.[10] If sustainable trust is to be achieved in order to not lose the focus on the goal of a Stratified Medicine, the complexity of the matter has to be taken into account and despite the possibly high financial and idealistic aid of resources; the risk of possible failure has to be mentioned. If, in spite of the possibly stony path, this vision (as a realistic one) shows better prospects compared to the current situation, this process can be of social value. So instead of promising a revolution and thereafter a rosy future in health care – as in the respective advertising brochures of the coalition for Personalized Medicine in America,[11] it is sufficient to assume that many

---

[10]   As an overview see: H. Braun, "Vertrauen als Ressource und als Problem.", in: *Die Neue Ordnung*, 62(4)/2008, p. 252-261.

[11]   See Personalized Medicine Coalition (Ed.), "The case for Personalized Medicine"; http://www.personalizedmedicinecoalition.org/sites/default/files/files/Case_for_PM_ 3rd_edition.pdf.

people will find it promising to believe that blockbuster medications could be differentiated into strongly, weakly and normally metabolizing and will be able to contribute to their development.[12] It is even possible that it will be motivating to push forward research by contributing to biobanks if it is a known fact that it is unsure whether the goal will be achieved and that its success even depends on the personal involvement. However, in order to make it possible to realistically achieve the goal of Stratified Medicine as well as to include the insight into a necessity of diverse personal and financial involvement and finally not to exclude the risk of failed expectations, this has to be eventually communicated in an evident, comprehensible and honest way. Too much unfulfilled trust has been invested in the field of human biotechnology over the last years, so that now, trust can probably only be won by respectively cautious strategies.

If deconstructing the current linguistic policies on the term of 'Individualized Medicine' does not discredit the matter itself, on the contrary there is important potential in the developmental dynamics of Stratified Medicine, which, however, is in need of an accompanying communication that is trust-building and realistic due to the matter, then such an extensive development implies ethical and socio-theoretical reflections. These will be addressed in the following trains of thought.

2 Ethical Questions for the So-Called Individualized Medicine

Turning towards the precise ethical challenges of the so-called Individualized Medicine while considering the deconstructive observations of linguistic policies; at first glance the following question arises: What can be ethically problematic concerning the development of a biomarker-based

---

[12] The figures of the latest Eurobarometer on the attitudes of the European population on biotechnologies can be read in this way: According to the Eurobarometer, after significantly raising the level of knowledge on the matter, almost half of the representatively questioned Europeans would be willing to donate data and samples for biobanks, which are required for a Stratified Medicine. See G. Gaskell, S. Stares, A. Allansdottir, N. Allum, P. Castro, Y. Esmer, C. Fischler, J. Jackson, N. Kronberger, J. Hampel, N. Mejlgaard, A. Quintanilha, A. Rammer, G. Revuelta, P. Stoneman, H. Torgersen, W. Wagner, "Europeans and Biotechnology in 2010. Winds of change?"; http://ec.europa.eu/research/science-society/document_library/pdf_06/europeans-biotechnology-in-2010_en.pdf.

medicine? When taking into account the four criteria of biomedical ethics, which are regarded as standards in most Western cultures – respect of autonomy, non-harm, doing good and justice – and I add: benefit[13] – there seem to be not only few conflicts when looking at the aimed-for vision of the so-called Individualized Medicine, but the vision even seems to be ethically worthwhile and realizing it seems to be almost imperative. Categorizing something as imperative is the strongest pro-argument offered by ethics that reflects moral attitudes of human actions and organizational decisions according to their justification ability. What speaks on behalf of such a normative advocacy of the so-called individual medicine is the fact that at least all dimensions of its ideal aimed-for vision, namely determining therapies more exactly, especially medication on the background of differing metabolizing, avoiding inadequate and harmful therapies as well as recognizing and avoiding health risks, which are due to nutrition or exposition, correspond to the mentioned criteria of supporting individual autonomy, the dictate of non-harm, the imperative of doing good as well as the increase of justice and social benefit (by decreasing the diseases that take a heavy toll on the population). At most, what evokes a socio-ethical discussion are the profit expectations of the pharmaceutical industry by Stratified Medicine, hoped for by some, feared by others and not even predicted by a third party – especially when regarding the mentioned criterion of justice: Will the often criticized bio-patenting be employed in the context of this biotechnological development?[14] Will the so-called Individualized Medicine increase the gap in health care – between the poor and the rich within developed countries and between those and the (yet) undeveloped countries? Shouldn't the resources that are invested in this biotechnology in society as a whole be rather spent on elementary health promotion than on biomedical high tech?[15] And finally it must be questioned in regard to the so-called ethics of allocation, which analyzes questions of justice concerning the distribution of scarce resources through experimental game hard cases: What

---

[13] T. L. Beauchamp, J. F. Childress (Eds.), *Principles of Biomedical Ethics*, [6]Oxford 2009.

[14] See the comprehensive study of I. Schneider (Ed.), *Das europäische Patentsystem: Wandel von Governance durch Parlamente und Zivilgesellschaft*, Frankfurt a. M./NY 2010.

[15] Especially the last point of criticism ignores the fact that in a society functionally differentiated political options cannot be converted directly into business decisions. Nevertheless this does not mean that all business decisions are legitimate.

would be the level of degree of probability, determined by predicative tests, which indicates if a therapy works with someone, that defines whether this person loses his or her right to the therapy (especially if shown that many others would profit from the money thus available)?

Regarding the fact that the first questions on justice address the relation between developed and less developed countries[16] and that the latter questions do not exclusively aim at the so-called Individualized Medicine but can refer to top health care in the developed countries in general, it cannot be denied that there is an enormous convergence of normative and evaluative criteria with the aimed-for vision of Stratified Medicine. Thus the question arises, whether anyone criticizes this idea and the attempts to realize it. Such critical opinions do exist. Here, Regine Kollek will be mentioned as representative of those who have reservations concerning the so-called Individualized Medicine. Her complaints are partly identical to the linguistic-policy deconstructions mentioned in part 1: The expectations of the so-called Individualized Medicine were too euphoric[17]. Furthermore it should be considered: "Die individuelle [sic!; PD] Medizin darf trotz aller Chancen und Möglichkeiten den Menschen nicht aus den Augen verlieren."[18] The individual(ized) medicine must not lose sight of the human being, despite all chances and possibilities. Among other things, this could happen when the doctor forgets that he or she should be the primary and actual partner of the patient in the fight for his/her health under the pressure of integrating more and more scientific-technical knowledge in his/her practice and thus being primarily determined by those standards. Eventually, Kollek shares the concern already mentioned that the so-called Individualized Medicine has the potential to intensify existing socio-economical inequalities within the health care system.[19]

---

[16] For an overview, see H. Hahn (Ed.), *Globale Gerechtigkeit: eine philosophische Einführung*, Frankfurt a. M./NY 2009.

[17] See *R. Kollek*, "Diskussion um Individualmedizin ist noch viel zu euphorisch.", in: *Deutsches Ärzteblatt*, 106(42)/2009, p. A 2071.

[18] R. Kollek, "Diskussion um Individualmedizin", p. A 2071.

[19] See R. Kollek, "Gesellschaftliche Aspekte der 'Individualisierten Medizin'. Beitrag zum 'Expertengespräch mit Diskussion des TAB-Zukunftsreports: Individualisierte Medizin und Gesundheitssystem'"; http://www.hf-initiative.de/fileadmin/dokumente/ProGesundheit_9_2009.pdf.

The points of criticism stated by Kollek have already been partly mentioned in the considerations so far and have been deemed remarkable – likewise the problematic, since hardly compliable euphoria concerning the so-called Individualized Medicine which is obviously controlled by interests of some. Other reservations seem to be comprehensible at a first glance but are hardly sustainable; on the contrary they prove to be ethically highly problematic themselves. The use of medical high technology, especially if improving health care lastingly, does not principally contradict to a relationship based on partnership between doctor and patient. On the contrary, good medical technology could even create space for an improved communication in this core of the medical system. The circumstance that this does not happen often is a social misallocation of resources, to be precise: it is health-politically wanted or accepted – at all means, this assumption becomes true when considering how important the dimension of face-to-face communication actually is, as well for the salutogenesis of the patients, as for the job satisfaction of those working in the health system (and thus for their state of health).[20] Nevertheless, all this said, there is no counterargument for abandoning medical research and technological progress. Instead, doctors have to be familiarized with new technologies and parameters have to be created, so that the talking medicine will still be valued more.

Beyond those points of criticism there is Kollek's and Lemke's unease, which is part of their reservations regarding biomarker-based medicine in general and genome-based medicine in particular, which they have been stating for many years.[21] Kollek and Lemke have supported the thesis that employing genome-based diagnostics would lead to the birth of the so-called person at genetic risk.[22] This person could be distinguished by three

---

[20] See T. Greenhalgh, B. Hurwitz, (Eds.), *Narrative-based Medicine – sprechende Medizin: Dialog und Diskurs im klinischen Alltag*, Bern 2005.

[21] See R. Kollek, T. Lemke (Ed.), *Der medizinische Blick in die Zukunft. Gesellschaftliche Implikationen prädiktiver Gentests*, Frankfurt a. M./NY 2008.

[22] See R. Kollek et al., *Der medizinische Blick in die Zukunft*, p. 150-160 and T. Lemke,"Von der sozialtechnokratischen zur selbstregulatorischen Prävention: Die Geburt der genetischen Risikoperson.", in: A. Hilbert, W. Rief, P. Dabrock (Eds.), *Gewichtige Gene. Adipositas zwischen Prädisposition und Eigenverantwortung*, Bern 2008, p. 151-165. In the main text I state parts of my contribution to this collected volume in which I critically deal with the theses of Kollek and Lemke among other things; see P. Dabrock, "Risikodimensionen genetischer Tests für Adipositas – sozialethische

elements: On the one hand, the figure of the "genetic fate" would be dismissed on behalf of a figure of increasing calculation forced upon the individual and of control over one's own genetically risky body; on the other hand, the consequence of this would mean deferring from an originally socio-economical relational prevention to a behavioral prevention depending on the individual's personal responsibility, which would orientate at their own genetically risky body equipment. Thirdly, this transition to a 'self-adjusting prevention' would leave the people in a 'nether land between health and disease'.[23] Therefore the individual would be more and more strongly identified with their own health, or more pointedly: Missing health would be stigmatized as self-inflicted without the individual possessing the respective resources of autonomous decision making and acting. All of the three developments are criticized by Lemke and Kollek as restricting freedom and often being socially unjust: Calculation and control over one's own bodily, especially genetic dispositions would only be possible to a minor degree in many cases; they would not create more freedom due to this hardly redeemable health autonomy, but they would restrict this freedom by the ever-present discrepancy between wanting and accomplishing. At this point – applying normative dynamics which are basically unrealizable while aiming at individual behavior – society[24] would deny its own responsibility to guaranty possible elementary circumstances and conditions for a healthy form of living. This exactly would be the claim of social justice.

3 Actual Ethical Perspectives Beyond General Suspicion and Uncritical Advocacy

Now, how to react in an actually socio-critical way to the outlined challenges of either exuberantly supporting the so-called Individualized

---

Perspektiven.", in: A. Hilbert, W. Rief, P. Dabrock (Eds.), *Gewichtige Gene. Adipositas zwischen Prädisposition und Eigenverantwortung*, Bern 2008, p. 173-198 (see for further literature).

[23] See T. Lemke, "Von der sozialtechnokratischen zur selbstregulatorischen Prävention", p. 157.

[24] What is to be understood by society is often not explained in social theories oriented on Foucault. Even a thesis like Luhmann's is not discussed, which claims that 'society' only exists as the limit-concept of the functional systems of politics, economics, law, religion etc., which have their own regularities.

Medicine or putting it under the general suspicion of promoting the terrifying vision of the person at genetic risk? On the level of prudence I have already pointed out that sustainable trust in an indeed promising but definite biotechnological development rather needs to be built on realistic than utopian visions. However, the ethical reflection does not stop at this level of reasoning. Therefore it would be problematic from an ethical perspective and not only by sage reasons to withdraw scarce financial and idealistic resources, which are possibly accessed via taxes, e.g. by governmental research at public research institutions, from competing projects and withhold them if it was clear that there was no or only very little potential in the so-called Individualized Medicine. Such an allocation would be ethically reprehensive as misallocation.

Beyond stating the avoidance of obvious misallocations as the minimum condition of ethical legitimation, it is necessary to assess the probability of the occurrence of its chances and risks against one-sided promotion or general criticism in order to be able to ethically judge the so-called Individualized Medicine. This risk assessment has to happen – adapting a well-known differentiation by Niklas Luhmann – in regard of time, matter and society. The question is: Who is when and to what extent affected of specific chances or risks and how can he/she handle such risks in a constructive way (or not)? The risk assessment of the so-called Individualized Medicine, which is sensitive to social ethics, thus takes into account the biotechnological probability as well as the social assessment (and its extrapolating transformations). While doing so, this assessment is not made in an abstract or speculative way but takes into account legal parameters which range from human rights standards via constitutional principles to simple legal norms. Such legal parameters are important for an actual ethical assessment of the so-called Individualized Medicine, because they help assessing whether certain visions, be they affirmative or critical, entail real consequences for society in the near future according to the Thomas theorem mentioned at the beginning or not.[25] Besides the scientific risk assessment and the determination of the potential of social conflicts, it is the

---

[25] Especially when assessing the concerned vision that the dispositif of a person of genetic risk can become true, this examination of the existing legal regulatory regime plays a significant role, which is to be proven.

analysis of the capacity of the existing regulating regime that belongs to the 'vision assessment'[26] of new technologies and biomedical trends.

On the background of the mentioned, actually ethical standards for an analysis concerning the vision of the person at genetic risk and its accompanying questioning of the so-called Individualized Medicine, it can be stated: On the surface, the feeling of fear, which appears if the trends outlined by Kollek and Lemke were true, is comprehensible. Thus it is crucial to ask if the conditions on which the trends and the thesis are founded are plausible themselves. This is, however, not the case. On the factual level the possible extent of intrusion of non-genetic biomarker tests into the way of living, one's own feeling of identity or possible discrimination and stigmatization is underestimated. A positive AIDS test can lead to graver consequences in all three dimensions than a hardly informative so-called genetic test for a multifactorial disease. Furthermore, the few genetic tests on classically segregating dispositions do not lead to general statements on genetic tests and the associated construction of a person at genetic risk. If nowadays people talk of the post-genomic era not only for scientific but also for research-policy reasons, the true core of this expression lies in the fact that the original expectations of genetics, which say it should discover and explain how *one* gene encodes *one* genetic product, are long outdated. In fact, it has to be taken into account that there are intra- and extra-organismic environments, behavior, nutrition and exposition influencing gene, extent and manifestation of genomic effects. If that is the case, the alleged risks that arise from the allegedly growing relevance of genomic knowledge not only for medicine but also for the actual way of living of the people must be put in context, i.e. they have to be conceived and classified as less important than before. Instead of prolonging an obsolete understanding of genetics into the future, the present level of information – that genomic knowledge is important for the medical progression but only to a certain extent and most of all that it is not exceptional – should be spread at schools, in the media and through other public channels of distribution. Since the effects that allegedly make it exceptional (great depth of intrusion, relevance for family relations and plans of reproducing, missing ability to correct) partly

---

[26] See J. Grin, A. Grunwald (Eds.), *Vision Assessment: shaping technology in 21st century society: towards a repertoire for technology assessment*, Wissenschaftsethik und Technikfolgenbeurteilung 4, Berlin/Heidelberg 2000.

apply to other biomarkers, too, and would have to be clearly differentiated by the respective kind of genetic test, it can only be spoken of the often stated specialty but not of the exceptionality of genetic knowledge. As a consequence for this side of the ethical assessment of the so-called Individualized Medicine it follows: If the knowledge on the significantly limited importance of the genome was conveyed to the channels of distribution of media, education, law, science and politics to a greater extent, the idea of being able to constantly influence one's own health by using genomic knowledge could be rejected as a travesty. It would be ethically reasonable to respectively enlighten people instead of perpetuating such a scientifically not verified exceptionalism by using dark visions of self-imposed diseases due to genetic knowledge.

Concerning the so-called Individualized Medicine, one should not ask for the ethical precariousness of specific methodical questions ("Are the possibilities of the so-called Individualized Medicine based on genetic tests or not? If yes, then the development as a whole has to be regarded critically."), but for the expectable physical, psychic and social extent of intrusion into a person's present and future way of life – no matter which method has been used to achieve it. The user's psychological and social problems concerning the possibilities of the so-called Individualized Medicine and thus its ethical assessment depend on such expectations and the fulfillment of such expectations.

Such an analysis of the extent of intrusion does not take place in an empty space but can rest upon established standards of human and civil rights, often in terms of a written constitution – at least in Germany, Europe and most of the developed countries. Discriminations due to genetic characteristics or disabilities – no matter how they are diagnosed or where they originate from – are legally condemned by the UN, the European anti-discrimination policy and the German *Grundgesetz* and the simple law of genetic diagnostics. Admittedly, it is true that it has to be thoroughly observed, if a mindset is spreading in society under the surface which runs contrary to this unanimous and decisive normative framework and eventually subverts[27] it, and if it has to be intervened as the case may be. If this

---

[27] The movie GATTACA (written and directed by Andrew Niccol, USA 1997) shows in an impressive way how in "the not too distant future", as it is said at the beginning of the movie, discrimination against people with genetic characteristics, regarded as

was necessary and the normative entities wanted to counteract, which was justified by the tradition of preserving the human rights, there would have to be some advance on different channels which would have to be made up of increased enlightenment, legal protective regimes and stimuli for avoiding the threat of exclusion. However, the existing legal standards of protection and participation, which surely are in need of more solid strategies of implementation – as the attempts of realizing the so-called UN convention on the rights of persons with disabilities presently show – can be regarded as an important and at the time being stable cultural achievement, which dismisses any hasty and historically decaying dramatized vision of a regime of genetic discrimination into the realm of fantasy.

It is self-evident due to the *conditio humana,* which implies change and progress that the framework of interventions and thus their social consequences have to be re-considered due to the integration of knowledge based on biomarkers in clinics and public health care with the goal of therapy and more effective and efficient prevention with less negative side effects. Nevertheless, it has to be kept in mind what Novas and Rose matter-of-factly add for consideration: "We shall argue that, far from generating resignation to fate or passivity in the face of biological destiny or bio-medical expertise, these new forms of subjectification are linked to the emergence of complex ethical technologies for the management of biological and social existence, located within a temporal field of 'life strategies', in which individuals seek to plan their present in the light of their beliefs about the future that their genetic endowment might hold. These new modes of subjectivity produce the obligation to calculate choices in a complex interpersonal field, not only in terms of individuals' relations to themselves, but also in terms of their relations to others, including not only actual and potential kin, past and present, but also genetic professionals and biomedical researchers."[28] Insofar as the respective self-conception of the persons acting is involved in such questions without any doubt ("Who do we want to be?"), changes that arise from the so-called Individualized Medicine have to be attended by ethics. Against the background of these new developments it has to be reckoned that – as Kollek and Lemke predict – the notions of 'health' and 'disease'

---

genetically pathological, can spread despite such legal norms.

[28] C. Novas, N. Rose, "Genetic risk and the birth of the somatic individual.", in: *Economy and Society*, 29(4)/2000, p. 485-513, p. 488.

will be redetermined. Actually, it would be not acceptable regarding ethical and legal aspects that persons in an intermediate state between prediction and (possible but not certain) onset of a disease would be treated on the one hand as non-invalids which are able to make completely autonomous decisions – when it comes to claims or benefit assignments – but on the other hand, as invalids they would be considered a risk for insurance companies or at work – when they wanted to claim their rights at those institutions. For pointing at such precarious constellations (at least as possible scenarios), the credit belongs to the works on the self-regulation of the person at genetic risk regarding Foucault's governmentality approach.[29] However, all of this should not be staged as a spectacle as the thesis of the person at genetic risk suggests, especially since normative legal and moral regimes of regulation, which are widely accepted, oppose to this pessimistic vision.

4 Continuation in the Medium and in the Long Run, (Not Only) from a Theological-Ethical Perspective

After outlining the immediate ethical challenges of the so-called Individualized Medicine beyond the critically considered linguistic policies and the equally dismissible exaggerated staging of concern, some fundamental questions on the self-conception of the human being, which the so-called Individualized Medicine, yet not exclusively, but progress in modern medicine in general entails, should be addressed eventually.

Firstly, the challenges which are waiting to be dealt with temporally, factually and socially in the medium run on the way to the development

---

[29] See R. Kollek, "Diskussion um Individualmedizin", p. 17; R. Kollek et. al., *Der medizinische Blick in die Zukunft*; T. Lemke,"Von der sozialtechnokratischen zur selbstregulatorischen Prävention"; P. Dabrock, "Risikodimensionen genetischer Tests für Adipositas– sozialethische Perspektiven". Apart from that: No one would want to summon the alternatives from which the critically interpreted self-regulation has developed: 'genetic fate' and 'medical paternalism'. The latter contradicts to the achievements of including elements of autonomy in the doctor-patient-relationship which was asymmetrical until far into the 20th century – not due to factually inappropriate reasons but also and most of all, because it was realized that a symmetric patient-therapist-relation is beneficial for medical success. It would be anachronistic romanticizing to focus further on the topos of 'genetic fate', which is left after dismissing the term 'person of genetic risk' as an alternative concept.

of the stratified or the so-called Individualized Medicine have to be considered: Before the effects of the so-called Individualized Medicine, which will still take some time to become real, can gain ground, extensive collections have to be made in order to gather person-related data concerning the medical history of the proband and his/her way of living (including nutrition and exposition to possibly harmful environmental influences). Such collections frequently exist – especially, but not exclusively, in Scandinavia – and they are partly arranged generically like the so-called UK Biobank, partly they focus on certain diseases or groups of diseases. At the moment, governance strategies of such biobank enterprises are being urged, not only nationally but also on a European and even global level, in order to be biomedically effective, seek a sufficient legal balance of regulation between the protection of the probands and the freedom of research, be socially responsible and economically efficient.[30] In doing so, those responsible are aware of the fact that such projects entail risks but also concerns, due to a general combination of enthusiasm for knowledge, alignment to the common good and simply self-interest.[31] The central issue is that probands or those who should be won over to take part in such research projects fear that their own data could be shared abusively, that they could be become known out of the original purpose of collecting and in the worst case even lead to discriminating or stigmatizing effects (with insurance companies or employers).

It is broadly agreed on the fact that those undeniable risks of biobank research, which represent the necessary step on the way to the aimed-for Stratified Medicine, can only be counteracted if the institutions involved develop a lastingly effective regime of trust – including the respect for privacy and possible transformations in the information age, ranging from Facebook to biobank companies.[32] In order to achieve the necessary level of trust, informed mechanisms of consent or contract must be established, transparency of the procedures of research must be practiced in regard to the probands and the general public. This includes firstly perceiving the asym-

---

[30] See http://www.bbmri.eu and http://www.p3g.org.

[31] See H. Gottweis, A. R. Petersen (Eds.), *Biobanks: Governance in Comparative Perspective*, London/NY 2008.

[32] See http://www.private-gen.eu; the considerations presented here have been developed against the background of this research project.

metry of information and power between the research institutes and the probands and removing it as much as possible. Such efforts would include not only considering the probands as objects of science but as partners in the scientific process and thus considering appropriate forms of benefit-sharing (which do not have to consist of financial payment but could possibly be realized as indirect engagement in educational measures in the context of research).[33] Furthermore, such standards of transparency, building trust and appreciation of the probands have to be generated from the respective cultural and regional characteristics and cannot be deduced from an abstractly universal perspective – as empirical studies and normative considerations prove.[34]

The statement "Human-Biobanks for Research" of the German Ethics Council[35] works with a so-called five-pillar model towards exactly such an extensive governance strategy backing on institutional trust. The especially strong pillar of trust in biobank-secrecy, which is meant to extent the doctor-patient confidentiality to all persons working in the biobank process, is surrounded by organizational suggestions for determining the use allowed, for including ethics commissions, for quality management and for mechanisms of transparency. By not following just one strategy but by relying on pillars supporting each other, the German Ethics Council causes the impression that a "house of trust" is well founded in order to adequately confront the complex challenges and risks of the biobank research in principle. This house built on such pillars has to be filled with life in order to truly become "house of trust". That means that on the other hand, the respective biobank projects have to permanently subject their own matter-specific but also communicative activities to a critical monitoring. If this is the case, there is hope that the regulating regimes already established for the protection against genetic discrimination, which will hopefully soon be extended to discriminations resulting from other biomarkers, will be filled with life.

---

[33] For those quality criteria inducing trust see especially the joint final statement of the participants of the conference "Trust in Biobanking" 2008 in Marburg; documented in: P. Dabrock, J. Ried, J. Taupitz (Eds.), *Trust in Biobanking: Dealing with Ethical, Legal and Social Issues in an Emerging Field of Biotechnology*, Berlin/Heidelberg 2012.

[34] M. Häyry, R. Chadwick, V. Árnason, G. Árnason (Eds.), *The Ethics and Governance of Human Genetic Databases: European Perspectives*, Cambridge 2007.

[35] See Deutscher Ethikrat (Ed.), *Humanbiobanken für die Forschung. Stellungnahme*, Berlin 2010.

Beyond such actually ethical and legal perspectives in the medium run, there are also long-run questions that must be publicly debated regarding but not exclusively founding on the developments of the so-called Individualized Medicine. They concern the human self-conception in one's limitedness as well as one's eligible pursuit of treating one's body responsibly and thus promoting health and fighting diseases: What do we expect from medicine? What is it able to do and what not? Does it take over the function of a salvation vision because life is understood as the "last chance"[36] and thus it has to be preserved at all costs as long as possible? But how is this function realized? Is it sufficient to have the idea of a medicine that more strongly relies on biotechnological developments (even through the respective systems of compensation and accounting) or to have the idea of a medicine that also allows communicative dimensions to play a constitutive role and does not end medical and nursing work at a point where a restitutio ad optimum or ad integrum is no longer within sight? How is such medical progress to be financed? Which other medical or nursing alternatives, which other public goods are possibly neglected if proportionally plenty of funds are put into this field of research? On the other hand it has to be asked: Which disadvantages concerning innovations and national economy will arise if a major trend in medical development will not be taken up and proactively promoted in a country otherwise established in the field of high technology? Finally: How will the respective understanding of the social guiding principles 'autonomy', 'solidarity', 'justice', 'community', 'standardization' and 'normality', also in their mutual relationships, be changed by the possible focus on (which version of) the so-called Individualized Medicine?

From the perspective of the religious and cultural tradition of Christianity and its theological reflection, at least the following suggestions can be put forward to the discourse on the progress of medical knowledge and its growing integration into the lives of human beings, which thus directly refer to the so-called Individualized Medicine: Christianity, especially in its Protestant coining, regards the human being as being in a form of responsibility limited by God and precisely by this limitation in a relieving and thus strengthened responsibility, above all, for others (to put it in classical terms:

---

[36] See M. Gronemeyer, *Das Leben als letzte Gelegenheit.*

it regards the human being as meant for brotherly love). This understanding of life in its reconciled limitedness achieves a fundamentally positive attitude towards healing diseases, since on the one hand, it can appreciate the body as the temple of the Holy Spirit (1 Cor 6:19) and thus can give respective care and nursing. On the other hand, this concern is not overextended due to the limitedness of all life regarding God, so that a kind of religion of the body would be enforced. Within the world this life is also the "last chance" from a Christian perspective, however this world is not – from a Christian perspective – God's last chance for the human being. Therefore expectations of salvation are not related to the medical progression. However, a general condemnation has to be dismissed either. Thus, the progress of medicine, including the so-called Individualized Medicine, should not be simply rejected, on the contrary it can be regarded with favor.

However, the limited favor towards medical progress is bound to certain criteria due to the mentioned perspective of reconciled limitedness: Ex negativo, the hope of achieving security in life with the help of biomarker-based medicine[37] is rejected. Christian faith confronts the belief in achieving meaning in life in a way as risk-free and as self-confident as possible by technology with the trust in ultimately being carried by God without having to refuse insurances, risk precaution and fighting life-threatening or life-restricting suffering in the penultimate. However, they belong to this penultimate realm, not to the last realm of the determination of the meaning of life. After all, Christianity – and perhaps this was an important factor of its groundbreaking attractiveness in the religiously pluralistic antique society – has always put healing efforts in the context of communicative atten-

---

[37] Hardly any other book does inform about the ambivalent effects of genomic knowledge on the bodily self-conception of the modern human being in such a brief and eloquent form as the report by the well-known novelist Richard Powers about his experience on having his genome analyzed, see R. Powers (Ed.), *Das Buch Ich #9: eine Reportage*, Frankfurt a. M. 2010. Paradigmatically, some especially impressive quotes will be mentioned here which emphasize his being drawn back and forth between enthusiasm for the new possibilities and profound skepticism, especially in such a composition: "Wenn man es ganz aufs Wesentliche reduziert, geht es beim individuellen Genom um Kontrolle." (p. 61), "Ich bin ein neuer Mensch geworden." (p. 76), "Ich selbst hingegen werde mich wohl nie wieder vollkommen sicher fühlen." (p. 55), "Es heißt ja, die Wahrheit solle uns befreien. Doch ein immer größeres Wissen erweist sich auch als immer kürzere Leine." (p. 59).

Peter Dabrock

tion to the sick and the needy and it has vice versa not understood nursing from the point of view of the medical task. Motivated not only but also by the Judgment speech in Matthew 25:31-46, which tells about the possibility of meeting Christ in any sick person, elements of medicine, nursing and dialog are mutually linked. If this is true, then ideal Christian life praxis and theory on leading life strengthens the irritation mentioned in the first chapter that truly Individualized Medicine would be that kind of medicine that saw the individual as individual, i.e. in his/her personality and not only in his/her individual genomic manifestation. In order to turn this irritation into something constructive: When medicine becomes based on biomarkers but truly keeps the *whole* human being as a person in mind, beyond the stratifying precision of therapies, then it is an important contribution to truly Individualized Medicine.

Those medical procedures which are labeled with the term "Individualized Medicine", which remains to be considered in a critical way, should not exclude anyone according to the Christian tradition. The Judgment speech in Matthew 25 again points paradigmatically at that, though it is not exclusive in the biblical tradition and the religio-cultural practice of Christianity: "Whatever you did for one of the least of these brothers of mine, you did for me." (Mt 25:40)[38] Accordingly, the credibility of the promise of "individualized" medicine has to prove itself for the socio-ethical doctrine of Christianity, which calls this devotion to the weak and the oppressed the "primary option for the disadvantaged ones" and for which they can claim a high convergence to present theories of justice with their general impetus of inclusion based on human rights, and show if it will lead to reducing inequalities concerning health. It significantly and sustainably influences – according to established epidemiological knowledge – the fair equality of opportunities. This, on the other hand, forms the foundation of the broadly agreed-upon socio-theoretical promise of the Western doctrine of freedom. Where there is freedom founded in such a way that all, including the weakest, are able to really participate in social communication,[39] possibly even by means of the so-called Individualized Medicine, there the call for more

---

[38] It would be a church-centric misunderstanding if "brothers" was identified only as church members.

[39] See P. Dabrock (Ed.), *Befähigungsgerechtigkeit: ein Grundkonzept konkreter Ethik in fundamentaltheologischer Perspektive*, Gütersloh 2011.

autonomy in the health system may be made. Nevertheless, it corresponds to the orientation of the theories of justice and solidarity of Christian social ethics that – mostly by sufficient efforts in the field of education – such ability is intensively prepared and realized by differentiations in class, gender and ethnicity. If only claimed pro forma, the otherwise legitimate call for autonomy loses its ethical justification. Contrary to that, all efforts that aim at achieving the empowerment of each individual are approved of from a perspective of social ethics. If an Individualized Medicine managed to contribute to this core of Western culture because it promotes health for preferably everyone by a more precise therapy, it would be approved of. In order for this to come true, its protagonists should pay attention to the concerns of linguistic policies, to the corridors of social ethics and law and to the questions coming from the Christian tradition. If this happens, the trust in the new trend of medical procedures can grow. This could be worth it.

Personalized Medicine as Encouragement and Discouragement of Patient Autonomy

Diana AURENQUE

Abstract: The concept of "Personalized Medicine" is clearly focused on the patient. This patient orientation should contribute to an increase of accuracy and efficiency of therapeutic, preventive or rehabilitative interventions. Against this background, it has been argued that Personalized Medicine promotes respect for patient autonomy. In this paper, I will focus on the relationship between Personalized Medicine and the autonomy of patients/individuals in terms of its concrete bioethical implications. I will argue that Personalized Medicine can be understood not only as encouragement but also as discouragement of patient autonomy. In the first part of this paper, I will introduce the concept of Personalized Medicine and discuss the importance of the concept of autonomy within the philosophical tradition as well as in the current medical-ethical discourse, especially in Beauchamp's and Childress' principlism. Furthermore I will expose that there are reasons to understand Personalized Medicine as an encouragement of patient autonomy. The active role of patients in decisions and actions regarding their health care is a strong argument in favor of patient autonomy. On the other hand, I also argue that as a result of the medical tools of Personalized Medicine (such as the use of genome testing and online resources) it may threaten patient autonomy. Finally, I will argue that Personalized Medicine deserves a careful ethical discussion in view of this paradoxical situation and I will outline some consequences of this issue.

1 Introduction

The concept of "Personalized Medicine" is clearly focused on the patient. This patient orientation should contribute to increase the accuracy and efficiency of therapeutic, preventive or rehabilitative interventions. Against this background, it has been argued that Personalized Medicine promotes respect for patient autonomy. In this paper, I will focus on the relationship between Personalized Medicine and the autonomy of patients/individuals in terms of its concrete bioethical implications. I will argue that Personalized Medicine can be understood not only as encouragement but also as discouragement of a patient's autonomy. In the first part of this paper, I will introduce the concept of Personalized Medicine after which I will go on to discuss the importance of the concept of autonomy in the philosophical tradition as well as in the current discourse within the field of medical ethics, with an emphasis on Beauchamp's and Childress' principlism. Then, I will demonstrate that there are reasons to understand Personalized Medicine as an encouragement of patient autonomy. The active role of patients in decisions and actions regarding their health care is a strong argument in favor of the autonomy of patients. On the other hand, I also argue that as a result of the medical tools it offers (such as the use of genome testing and online resources) Personalized Medicine may threaten patient autonomy. Finally, I will argue that Personalized Medicine deserves a careful ethical discussion in view of this paradoxical situation and I will outline some consequences of this issue.

2 What is Personalized Medicine? Between concept and reality

In recent years, there has been a heated discussion about the concept of Personalized Medicine and Personalized Health Care. This growing interest is due to the fact that medical researchers are becoming more and more convinced that the variability in patients' responses to treatments is strongly connected to their specific genetic constitution and variability. Therefore, new genomic technologies, like genomic biomarker signatures of disease, are being developed. Many potential benefits are expected from the development of Personalized Medicine: patients' responses to therapies and drugs could be predicted more accurately so that side effects could be reduced and health care generally improved; patients would have more personal involvement in the decision-making process concerning their treatments; Personalized Health Care would reduce the likelihood of wrong diagnoses and treatments of diseases so that patients could save money, etc.

The exact meaning of Personalized Medicine is controversial. As L. J. Lesko from the U.S. Food and Drug Administration (FDA) states, there is no single, dominant definition of Personalized Medicine: "The most common vision of PM [Personalized Medicine] is that drugs and drug doses are made safer and more effective because they are chosen according to an individual's genetic makeup."[1] Therefore, targeted therapies for patients as well

---

[1] L. J. Lesko, "Personalized Medicine: Elusive Dream or Imminent Reality?", in: *Clinical Pharmacology & Therapeutics*, 81(6)/2007, p. 807-816, p. 809.

as targeted doses of medication are two essential components of Personalized Medicine.[2] It predicts the end of the "one size fits all" dosing model of medicine as well as the end of the trial-and-error method of prescribing of medication. A broader definition is provided by the U.S. Personalized Medicine Coalition: "Some have suggested that Personalized Medicine is the application of genomic data to better target the delivery of medical interventions. Others have suggested that it is a crucial tool in the discovery and clinical testing of new products. And others have suggested that it involves the application of sophisticated, clinically useful diagnostic tools that may help determine a patient's predisposition to a particular disease or condition. In fact, personalized medicine can encompass all of those concepts."[3]

Personalized Medicine is an emerging field of clinical practice in which the use of molecular (i.e. genetic) data plays an important role. However, genetic information is just one among a plethora of data that is relevant for such medicine. For that reason, Personalized Medicine also represents a strong connection between new biological knowledge and new information tools (such as the internet).[4] The use of a lot of non-genetic data such as demographic information, study and clinical observations of diseases as well as environmental factors and dietary habits are crucial for the accuracy of personalized diagnoses and treatments of patients.

Although the concept of Personalized Medicine has already established itself in the public sphere, its reality has yet to be settled. Some institutions like the *Personalized Medicine Coalition,* are very enthusiastic and convinced that Personalized Medicine is a "new healthcare paradigm with far-reaching implications".[5] Others are more cautious and claim that Personalized Medicine should actually be understood as a "paradigm that exists more in conceptual terms than in reality"[6]. There are only "a few marketed

---

[2]   See L. J. Lesko, "Personalized Medicine", p. 809.

[3]   Personalized Medicine Coalition, "Personalized Medicine Coalition Mission and Principles"; http://www.personalizedmedicinecoalition.org/sites/default/files/pmc_mission-principles.pdf, accessed November 25, 2012.

[4]   See U. S. Department of Human Health and Human Services (HHS) (Ed.), *Personalized Health Care: Pioneers, Partnerships, Progress*, Washington DC 2008, p. 10-11., accessed November 25, 2012.

[5]   http://www.personalizedmedicinecoalition.org/about/about-personalized-medicine/personalized-medicine-101/challenges, accessed November 25, 2012.

[6]   L. J. Lesko, "Personalized Medicine", p. 807.

drug-test companion products" to date, and clinical practices are not "set up to personalize medicine in the way that supporters have intended".[7] The U.S. leaders of the National Institutes of Health (NIH) and the Food and Drug Administration (FDA) are therefore committed "to help make Personalized Medicine a reality"[8] with the purpose of finding "the best ways to develop new therapies and optimize prescribing by steering patients to the right drug at the right dose at the right time."[9] For instance, with personal pharmacogenetic profiling it is possible to evaluate the individual efficacy of pharmacogenomics (like the anticoagulant "warfarin") and find the most suitable pharmacotherapy for each patient.

Regarding its practice, Personalized Medicine is actually Stratified Medicine, i.e. drugs or therapies are not being developed for individual people but for groups of people or medicines. Therefore, the following definition of Personalized Medicine was proposed by the U.S. President's Council of Advisors on Science and Technology (PCAST) in its report *Priorities for Personalized Medicine*: "'Personalized Medicine' refers to the tailoring of medical treatment to the individual characteristics of each patient. It does not literally mean the creation of drugs or medical devices that are unique to a patient, but rather the ability to classify individuals into subpopulations that differ in their susceptibility to a particular disease or their response to a specific treatment."[10] But even though it is controversial to what extent Personalized Medicine is actually a reality, there is no doubt that at least under those conditions, it is becoming one.[11]

Diagnostic testing is crucial for Personalized Medicine. Important instruments for such diagnostic testing are genetic tests. Today, genetic tests

[7] L. J. Lesko, "Personalized Medicine", p. 807.
[8] M. A. Hamburg, F. S. Collins, "The Path to Personalized Medicine", in: *The New England Journal of Medicine*, 363/2010, p. 301-304, p. 304.
[9] M. A. Hamburg et al., "The Path to Personalized Medicine", p. 1.
[10] President's Council of Advisors on Science and Technology (PCAST) (Ed.), *Priorities for Personalized Medicine*, Washington DC 2008, p. 1.
[11] Personalized medicine is rapidly becoming a reality, as Lesko says, "because of the increased awareness of the shortcomings in the delivery of drugs with adequate benefit/risk to patients, a better molecular understanding of how to optimize drug selection and dosing, and an increased demand for integrating more clinically relevant genetic information into the drug development process to improve both innovation and productivity" (L. J. Lesko, "Personalized Medicine", p. 807).

are used to predict the susceptibility of individuals to some drugs and diseases through the screening of a set of specific genes. Different genetic tests are used to detect monogenic diseases for common multifactorial diseases as well as for non-medical traits.[12] Biomarkers and tests are available for the identification and treatment of some forms of cancer (breast cancer, colon cancer or leukemia), cardiovascular disease, HIV, and other orphan diseases.[13] But as Jean-Jacques Cassiman in the EFGCP Annual Conference 2010 stated: "There is nothing for common diseases that could be commercialized sensibly."[14]

Personalized Medicine is a wide-ranging concept that is now becoming a reality. New treatments and diagnostics developments, such as personal genetic profiling for individual susceptibility to drugs and diseases as well as 'online medicine'[15], are considered mechanisms of a new age of Personalized Medicine.[16] There are significant reasons to understand these new technologies as an encouragement of the patient autonomy. Paradoxically, we will also see these technologies as being a contributing factor in discouraging patient autonomy. However, in order to reach this point, we must first recognize the importance of the principle of respect for autonomy in biomedical ethics.

---

[12] P. Borry, M. C. Cornel, H. C. Howard, "Where are you going, where have you been: a recent history of the direct-to-consumer genetic testing market", in: *Journal of Community Genetics*, 1(3)/2010, p. 101-106.

[13] A list is given by the U.S. Coalition for Personalized Medicine. See Personalized Medicine Coalition, "The case for Personalized Medicine"; http://www.personalizedmedicinecoalition.org/sites/default/files/files/Case_for_PM_3rd_edition.pdf, accessed November 25, 2012.

[14] European Forum for Good Clinical Practice Report (EFGCP) (Ed.), *EFGCP Annual Conference 2010. Aspects of Personalized Medicine for Society – A Challenge Yet to be Met*, Brussels 2010, p. 5.

[15] I understand 'online medicine' in terms of the definition by the Nuffield Council, namely as "developments in digital technology, largely involving the internet, that offer new ways for individuals to obtain and share health advice, diagnosis and medication, and which provides new possibilities for storing, accessing and sharing health records, monitoring the health status of individuals and communicating with health professionals and other patients." (Nuffield Council on Bioethics (Ed.), *Medical profiling and online medicine: the ethics of 'personalized healthcare' in a consumer age*, London 2010, p. xvii).

[16] See Nuffield Council on Bioethics, *Medical profiling and online medicine.*

3 The principle of respect for autonomy in the context of biomedical ethics

It has been said that Personalized Medicine contributes to a "consolidation of patient autonomy" and of their "sovereignty as consumers".[17] The respect for the autonomy of patients is a crucial ethical principle in modern biomedical ethics. However, this principle was not part of the Hippocratic Oath. The ethical principle of autonomy was implicitly introduced in the Nuremberg Codex under the word "consent" and later specified as "informed consent" by the Declaration of Helsinki (1964).[18] In the so-called *Belmont Report*[19] created by the National Commission for the Protection of Human Subjects of Biomedical and Behavioral Research in the late 70s, the respect for patient autonomy was explicitly connected with informed consent. This report had the purpose of providing a set of regulations for the protection of patients and human subjects in medical treatments and clinical trials, which proved to be extremely necessary after the controversial Tuskegee Syphilis Study (1932-1972). The introduction of autonomy as an ethical principle also intended to protect patients from the threat of paternalistic attitudes of physicians. Since then, the principle of respect for autonomy has become one of the most important ethical concepts in medical ethics.

But what does the word "autonomy" mean? Autonomy is not easy to define, because there are many different concepts related to it. Some of them are voluntariness or liberty, self-determination, independence, agency, integrity and responsibility as well as dignity. If we attend to the Greek etymology of the word "autonomy", this concept means that one gives oneself his or her own law, i.e. self-government. When we respect the autonomy of people, we respect the ways in which people govern their lives without trying to limit their self-government. With that in mind, it is not surprising

17 B. Hüsing, J. Hartig, B. Bührlen, T. Reiß, S. Gaisser (Ed.), *Individualisierte Medizin und Gesundheitssystem*, TAB-Arbeitsbericht 126, Berlin 2008.
18 World Medical Association (WMA) (Ed.), *WMA Declaration of Helsinki – Ethical Principles for Medical Research Involving Human Subjects*, Seoul 2008.
19 The National Commission for the Protection of Human Subjects of Biomedical and Behavioral Research, "The Belmont Report. Ethical Principles and Guidelines for the Protection of Human Subjects of Biomedical and Behavioral Research"; http://ohsr.od.nih.gov/guidelines/belmont.html, accessed November 25, 2012.

that autonomy was one of the most central concepts of the Enlightenment. In matters of ethics, autonomy represents the modern idea of a "moral consciousness of freedom", i.e. the responsibility of human beings to set norms is assumed as a vital and unquestionable condition for normative obligations.[20] Although there are different ways to legitimate autonomy, Kant's moral philosophy represents one of the most important accounts on this issue. According to Kant, the moral obligation of values or principles is grounded in the moral will or "good will" of human beings. However, the will is not always a good will: only if the will acts in accord with practical reason, i.e. the law that a human being gives himself through practical reason (as a categorical imperative and not for mere arbitrary reasons), does a moral law possess the character of a universal duty. Kant shows that autonomy can only be an ethical duty if this concept is understood as the possibility to make choices that are bound by one's own faculty of making moral law, which is to say they are justified by the claim of universal validity.[21] Furthermore, by recognizing the universal moral law of practical reason (as a categorical imperative) it is possible to become aware of not only the autonomy of human beings but also their own dignity as moral individuals.[22]

However, the most popular and widespread understanding of autonomy in medical bioethics is not Kantian but rather equivalent to fulfilling the requirements of informed consent, i.e. making free and informed decisions. According to this claim, autonomy assumes that patients have the cognitive capacity to understand their own situation and are able to make decisions concerning their care based on this understanding without being manipu-

---

[20] See M. Düwell, C. Hübenthal, M. H. Werner (Eds.), *Handbuch Ethik*, [2]Stuttgart/Weimar 2006, p. 311.

[21] See "Der Wille wird also nicht lediglich dem Gesetze unterworfen, sondern so unterworfen, daß er auch *als gesetzgebend* und eben um deswillen allererst dem Gesetze (davon er selbst sich als Urheber betrachten kann) unterworfen angesehen werden muß." (I. Kant, *Grundlegung zur Methaphysik der Sitten*. Edited by Tradition [2011], Riga 1785, p. 70f.)

[22] See I. Kant, *Grundlegung zur Methaphysik der Sitten*, p. 48: "Der Mensch, und überhaupt jedes vernünftige Wesen, existiert als Zweck an sich selbst, nicht bloß als Mittel zum beliebigen Gebrauche für diesen oder jenen Willen, sondern muß in allen seinen, sowohl auf sich selbst, als auch auf andere vernünftige Wesen gerichteten Handlungen jederzeit zugleich als Zweck betrachtet werden".

lated by others. In Beauchamp's and Childress' ethical approach *The Principle of Biomedical Ethics*[23], the most important work in biomedical ethics to date, autonomy is mostly understood in these terms.

According to Beauchamp's and Childress' principlism, the respect for autonomy is just one ethical principle among many, such as beneficence, nonmaleficence and justice. The authors' emphasis on the principle of autonomy is often misunderstood as if this principle were more highly recognized than the other principles. In the preface to the 6th edition of their book, Beauchamp and Childress argue against this misguided interpretation: "We have always argued that competing moral considerations validly override this principle under many conditions."[24] In accordance with this approach, clinicians consider the four principles as guiding of their actions in situations of ethical conflict. Beauchamp and Childress emphasize the *prima facie* validity of the principles, which means that under certain circumstances competing moral considerations override one or more principles. Beauchamp's and Childress' ethical principles are not founded in a moral theory with the claim of universal validity, but rather on the validity that these principles have in "common morality"[25].

Beauchamp and Childress understand the principle of respect for autonomy first and foremost as "respect for autonomous choices"[26], even though they recognize that autonomy is not all about autonomous choices.[27] The binding force of the principle of autonomy (understood as the respect for patients' autonomous choices) mostly appears in two different ways: as a "*negative* obligation", which means that a person is free from being coerced or manipulated by others into making autonomous choices; and as a "*positive* obligation", which means that a person is capable of making their own decision by having information disclosed and choices available.[28] The

---

[23] T. L. Beauchamp, J. F. Childress (Eds.), *Principles of Biomedical Ethics*, [6]Oxford 2009, p. 99-148.

[24] T. L. Beauchamp et al., *Principles of Biomedical Ethics*, p. 99: "Although we begin our discussion of principles of biomedical ethics with respect for autonomy, our order of presentation does not imply that this principle has moral priority over other principles. We do not hold, as some critics suggest, that the principle of respect for autonomy overrides all other moral considerations".

[25] T. L. Beauchamp et al., *Principles of Biomedical Ethics*, p. 99.

[26] T. L. Beauchamp et al., *Principles of Biomedical Ethics*, p. 99.

[27] See. T. L. Beauchamp et al., *Principles of Biomedical Ethics*, p. 100.

capacity for intentional action, known as "agency"[29], is also essential for autonomous actions. Beauchamp and Childress see different grades in which a choice can be described as an autonomous choice: It depends upon how *intentional*, how *informed* and how *free from external control* the choice was.[30] These three criteria should be taken into consideration while investigating to what extent an action can be described as an autonomous choice without the expectation of reaching an ideal degree of autonomy.[31] "Such consequential decisions must be *substantially* autonomous, but being *fully* autonomous is a mythical idea."[32] For Beauchamp and Childress, clinicians can actively contribute to the process of autonomous decision-making by patients by following different moral rules such as being honest or respectful of the privacy of others.[33]

A central aspect of autonomy refers to the *capacity* for autonomous choices. For this reason, some emphasize that autonomy is based on certain cognitive capacities that make it possible to act autonomously.[34] In Beauchamp's and Childress' ethics, this capacity is understood as "competence in decision making" and related to the "validity of consent".[35] Individuals are competent to make autonomous decisions, "if they have the capacity to understand the material information, to make a judgment about this information in light of their values, to intend a certain outcome, and to communicate freely their wishes to caregivers or investigators."[36] In this characterization of competence, there are many standards to be considered in order to decide how autonomous a choice may be. Among them are the ability to communicate a preference or choice, to comprehend one's situa-

---

[28] T. L. Beauchamp et al., *Principles of Biomedical Ethics*, p. 104.

[29] T. L. Beauchamp et al., *Principles of Biomedical Ethics*, p. 100.

[30] See T. L. Beauchamp et al., *Principles of Biomedical Ethics*, p. 101.

[31] See T. L. Beauchamp et al., *Principles of Biomedical Ethics*, p. 101.

[32] T. L. Beauchamp et al., *Principles of Biomedical Ethics*, p. 102.

[33] T. L. Beauchamp et al., *Principles of Biomedical Ethics*, p 104.

[34] Peter Singer for instance understands autonomy as a capacity of rational and self-conscious beings: "By 'autonomy' is meant the capacity to choose, to make and act on one's own decisions. Rational and self-conscious beings presumably have this ability, whereas beings who cannot consider the alternatives open to them are not capable of choosing in the required sense and hence cannot be autonomous" (P. Singer (Ed.), *Writings on an Ethical Life*, NY 2000, p.137).

[35] T. L. Beauchamp et al., *Principles of Biomedical Ethics*, p. 111.

[36] T. L. Beauchamp et al., *Principles of Biomedical Ethics*, p. 113.

tion and to understand relevant information as well as the ability of rational thought. If someone gives their consent to a particular medical procedure, the moral validity of this consent should initially evaluate the level of competence of this person. Without a certain level of competence, we cannot expect subjects to act autonomously and willingly take responsibility for their choices. Even if Beauchamp and Childress do not explicitly discuss this, a crucial way to legitimate the respect for patient autonomy is the fact that the attribution of responsibility is strongly connected to the ability to make free choices.[37]

Furthermore, giving consent as an autonomous act implies first of all the disclosure of information. This disclosure plays "a pivotal role"[38] in informed consent. Only on the basis of an adequate disclosure of information can patients be in a position to reflect on possible consequences, harms and benefits that their choices may have.

4 Encouragement of autonomy: more information, responsibility and voluntariness

Disclosure of information is one central standard in making autonomous choices. As we have seen, this disclosure implies that information can be available to individuals. Therefore, by improving the access to health-care information autonomy will be indirectly encouraged. The incorporation of new information tools via the internet, such as electronic health records (EHR) like that of MyGeisinger or health care websites have been considered a fundamental step in achieving Personalized Medicine. "Online Medicine" now makes a wide array of health care accessible to patients. This can also improve competence in decision making of individuals, inasmuch as additional information allows patients to have a better understanding of their respective situations.

This new technology also means a considerable change in the traditional relationship between patients and clinicians. A fundamental aspect of the traditional relationship between patients and clinicians is based on the assumption of a structural "information asymmetry"[39], which has impor-

---

[37] M. Düwell et. al., *Handbuch Ethik*, p. 545.
[38] T. L. Beauchamp et al., *Principles of Biomedical Ethics*, p. 121.
[39] Nuffield Council on Bioethics, *Medical profiling and online medicine,* p. 41.

tant ethical consequences for physicians: for a successful patient-clinician relationship, it is essential that patients have trust in not only the medical expertise but also the moral integrity of clinicians. In this asymmetrical relationship there is always the potential risk of physicians displaying paternalistic attitudes, in which patients' opinions about their own health play a secondary role while clinicians are the main authority and bear a major responsibility in the decision-making process. The new possibilities to access health-care information therefore imply a concrete way to increase the autonomy of patients. Using technologies like personal genetic profiling or online resources, individuals can access a wide spectrum of health-care information (diagnosis, prevention, medication, etc.) without having to go through a clinician. In such situations, the relationship between patients and clinicians clearly changes, as does their responsibility: patients become informed by their own means. They can also actively make decisions concerning the "management of their healthcare and health records" while assuming "more individual responsibility".[40]

Among other meanings, the word "personalized" can be understood as respect for the autonomy of patients in terms of respect for their own responsibility.[41] For the Nuffield Council, the new understanding of patient's responsibility in Personalized Medicine is part of the "responsabilisation"-movement. The process of responsabilisation of individuals concerning their health care attempts to reduce dependency and increase autonomy not only by granting individuals more rights, "but also obliging them to take greater responsibility for their own present and future health, welfare and security and that of their families and close communities, rather than allocating such responsibilities to an abstract 'society' or a distant state."[42] Patients should see themselves as part of a shared decision-making process, and they should actively participate in decisions regarding their own medical treatment.

The whole concept of Personalized Medicine is strongly connected to a "consumerist" understanding of health care. Some consider this "consumerist" turn to be the libertarian reply to the traditional "authoritarian"

---

[40]   Nuffield Council on Bioethics, *Medical profiling and online medicine*, p. 23.
[41]   See Nuffield Council on Bioethics, *Medical profiling and online medicine*, p. 30.
[42]   Nuffield Council on Bioethics, *Medical profiling and online medicine*, p. 39.

health care.[43] To view the patient-clinician relationship as a relationship between a consumer and a health care provider, has "the effect of democratizing the process of health care itself", [44] the U.S. Department of Health and Human Services has stated. Therefore, some say that patients should be seen "as partners" or also as "voters": "Patients could have a strong influence on the ethical and social implications of Personalized Medicine". [45]. In Personalized Medicine, patients are equally important as physicians in the process of decision-making: "The new patients could be more and more co-decision makers in their own health and in health policy".[46] According to this approach, patients can actively choose to assume more responsibility by seeking more information about their health care or by making their own free lifestyle choices. While the traditional patient is seen as a "passive recipient of information" who does not always fully comprehend his or her situation and therefore needs the authority of physicians, in Personalized Medicine individuals are seen as consumers who are "active" and "in control" of their situation. Accordingly, patients' decisions are oriented to their own needs and free from external or coercive control from clinicians.[47] Inasmuch as the consumer-supplier relationship is basically one of choice in which consumers can choose between different suppliers,[48] the introduction of a "consumerist"-model in health care increases the possibility of patients choosing the care that they desire.

5 Personalized Medicine as discouragement of autonomy

At the same time, the new forms of technology (personal genetic profiling and online medicine) can also be responsible for a discouragement of patient autonomy.

---

[43] Nuffield Council on Bioethics, *Medical profiling and online medicine*, p. 26.
[44] See HHS, *Personalized Health Care*, p. 11.
[45] EFGCP, *EFGCP Annual Conference 2010*, p. 9.
[46] EFGCP, *EFGCP Annual Conference 2010*, p. 9.
[47] See the report from the U.S. Department of Health and Human Services: "Our goal for PHM [Personalized Health Management] is to meet these needs by systematically eliciting information from consumers and by facilitating their ability to assume substantial decision responsibility and control" (HHS, *Personalized Health Care*, p. 10).
[48] See Nuffield Council on Bioethics, *Medical profiling and online medicine*, p.42.

The nearly limitless amount of information on the internet does not necessarily speak for its quality. The accuracy and reliability of the information on most websites about general health care and diseases, chat groups or other medical topics is not guaranteed, which means they can create needless confusion on various health-care matters. In addition, the risk of distributing misinformation can increase considerably. In a scenario full of misinformation patients can hardly make responsible and well-informed decisions. Furthermore, it is also questionable as to how free their decisions can be in such a context.

The information regarding personal genetic profiling may also be an obstacle for an autonomous choice. Some even claim that the most complex ethical, legal and social issues concerning personal genome testing refer to information.[49] Genetic or pharmacologic testing can not only provide relevant information about the matter for which the testing was conducted, but it also has the potential to reveal more genetic information than was initially intended. This risk is especially high in cases of non-targeted personal genome testing. This new situation involves ethical problems regarding the limit of volunteer consent to the extent that physicians cannot really counsel patients about possible outcomes, therapeutic options, or possible implications of their choices.

Genetic or pharmacology tests can help individuals to make autonomous choices only if the tests are reliable and accurate. New technologies in body imaging (a so-called "check-up" through computer tomography or magnetic resonance imaging) and DNA-testing are offered directly to consumers by commercial companies. Inasmuch as these tests are not always reliable or accurate, they can produce "false negatives or, more commonly, false positives, thereby creating needless confusion or anxiety."[50] Some of them can also "be medically or therapeutically meaningless, or of doubtful clinical validity and utility."[51] Therefore, these and other forms of technology should be evaluated by the European Medicines Evaluation Agency (EMEA) and the FDA first. However, it is known that the use of

---

[49] E. M. Bunnik, M. H. N. Schermer, A. Cecile, J.W. Janssens, "Personal genome testing: Test characteristics to clarify the discourse on ethical, legal and societal issues", in: *BMC Medical Ethics*, 12(11)/2011, p. 8.

[50] Nuffield Council on Bioethics, *Medical profiling and online medicine*, p. 25.

[51] Nuffield Council on Bioethics, *Medical profiling and online medicine*, p. 25.

new therapies, particularly in the USA, might guide clinical practice although the reliability of results from diagnostic tests has not been independently reviewed by the FDA.[52] Hamburg et al. report on an interesting example: "[I]n 2006, the FDA granted approval to rituximab (Rituxan) for use as part of first-line treatment in patients with certain cancers. Since then, a laboratory has marketed a test with the claim that it can distinguish the approximately 20% of patients who will not have a response to the drug from those who will. The FDA has not reviewed the scientific justification for this claim, but health care providers may use the test results to guide therapy."[53] The skepticism about the quality of some tests is also shared by European researchers.[54] Since health-care companies have mostly a financial interest in the development of new diagnostic and treatment tools, potential consumers should be skeptical about the many promises of Personalized Medicine.

Genetic testing offers a large amount of information that is not easy to understand. As Bunnik states, this information "may be too large for patients or consumers to process".[55] For autonomous choice, individuals must first be able to process the information that they receive in order to understand their situation. The correct understanding and interpretation of the genetic results is particularly important in the decision-making process. However, an additional problem arises. The correct use of genetic tests cannot guarantee accurate results: "Genetic tests are not perfect, in part because most gene mutations do not perfectly predict outcomes. Clinicians will need to understand the specificity and sensitivity of new diagnostics."[56] Clinicians must therefore also interpret the results of the genetic test with non-genetic factors in mind such as the patient's diet and environment, among other things. An excessive emphasis on genetic profiling could lead to a misunderstanding of the results of genome-based testing, inasmuch as pa-

---

[52] See. M. A. Hamburg et al., "The Path to Personalized Medicine", p. 2 f.

[53] M. A. Hamburg et al., "The Path to Personalized Medicine", p. 2 f.

[54] See EFGCP, *EFGCP Annual Conference 2010*, p. 6: "Many tests are implemented without proper evaluation of their clinical utility," said Corianne De Borgie from the Academic Medical Center of the University of Amsterdam. "We have a lot of diffusion of techniques, but many of them are not properly implemented or evaluated in patient care".

[55] E. M. Bunnik et al., "Personal genome testing", p. 4.

[56] M. A. Hamburg et al., "The Path to Personalized Medicine", p. 3.

tients may think that their genetic information is the only decisive factor to consider for health-care decisions. This contributes to a genetic determinism that threatens the very autonomy of the patient.

There are also ethical matters concerning the privacy of genetic data and other information about the patients: "there is also the risk that such technologies can be used to intrude on people's privacy in ways that may be unwelcome or not fully understood."[57] The same questions arise regarding the privacy of personal online records. Privacy and autonomy are related concepts: Patients have the right to decide whether they want to make their genetic or other medical data public. If the privacy of patients is not guaranteed, then their personal autonomy is in danger.

The increasing "responsabilisation" of individuals in Personalized Medicine may compromise the voluntariness of their decisions. First of all, there is the social risk that individuals who cannot or do not want to use new online technologies may become "second class citizens"[58] with the consequence that many of them feel a restriction on their liberties. As the Nuffield Council states, "the notion of responsibilisation through new technology raises important ethical issues as well, for example when individuals choose to reject rather than embrace such responsibility or when not all patient groups have equal access to the internet and its power of communication."[59] Personalized Medicine can therefore not only be seen as a possibility to encourage the autonomous acts of patients but also as an obligation. Personalized Medicine may be understood as the obligation of patients "to take a share of the responsibility" for health-care choices and its consequences. If this is the case, then it is also possible to believe that "[s]anctions or other consequences may flow from individuals not taking responsibility, either by not acting on the results of predictive tests, or perhaps, even by not informing themselves about their health risks."[60] In such a scenario, patients would probably take care of their health not as a matter of autonomous choice but because of guilt, fear of discrimination, fashion or other reasons. Moreover, the autonomous choice not to know about the

---

[57] Nuffield Council on Bioethics, *Medical profiling and online medicine*, p. 22.
[58] Nuffield Council on Bioethics, *Medical profiling and online medicine*, p. 22.
[59] See Nuffield Council on Bioethics, *Medical profiling and online medicine*, p. 39.
[60] Nuffield Council on Bioethics, *Medical profiling and online medicine*, p. 39.

future might make the patient "feel [...] condemned as irresponsible."[61] For example, if it is not only an expectation but also a duty for individuals to take care of their own health, it is theoretically possible that individuals who smoke, do not exercise on a regular basis or have unhealthy eating habits will not receive help from health-care providers.[62]

6 Conclusion

Ethical issues arise first, but not only, due to the leading role of autonomy in Personalized Medicine to the extent that this principle overrides other fundamental bioethical principles such as beneficence, nonmaleficence, and, above all, justice. Contrary to the widespread assumption that Personalized Medicine encourages the empowerment of individuals and their autonomy, we have reason to believe that Personalized Medicine may not contribute to diminish the autonomy of the individual. The ethical debate about Personalized Medicine should therefore cover not only the extent to which the principle of autonomy may be considered the highest principle in medicine, but also the extent to which patient autonomy is actually encouraged by Personalized Medicine. Personalized Medicine itself can actually put the principle of autonomy in jeopardy. Since the principle of respect for the autonomy of the patient is a central ethical principle in biomedical ethics and may be discouraged by Personalized Medicine, it is necessary to provide concrete recommendations for dealing with this situation.

One of the most important issues that can discourage autonomous choices is the large amount of information that individuals can obtain via online medicine and genetic profiling. The medical health information that individuals receive can have severe consequences for the management and control of their lifestyle and health-care decisions. Therefore, the use of new media technology like the internet in such a sensitive area as medicine must be taken into consideration not only in the context of biomedical ethics

---

[61] Nuffield Council on Bioethics, *Medical profiling and online medicine*, p. 39.

[62] Another example: "For example, the introduction of pharmacogenetics could lead to a further stratification of the market for medicines, discouraging pharmaceutical companies from developing medicines that would provide a significant benefit to only a small number of patients" (Nuffield Council on Bioethics (Ed.), *Pharmacogenetics: ethical issues*, London 2003, p. xiii).

but also in the wide context of media ethics. With the new possibilities of acquiring information through genetic testing and online medicine and the growing interest in these tools, we have to ask ourselves to what extent which information is valuable.

The selection of relevant information about health care is fundamental. However, it is just as difficult to define what "relevant information" might be as it is to set standards for it. In the case of genetic testing, we could only consider its "clinical utility", that is "the ability of a screening or diagnostic test to prevent or ameliorate adverse health outcomes such as mortality, morbidity, or disability through the adoption of efficacious treatments conditioned on test results",[63] as a standard to identify relevant information. In this case, genetic information is only relevant if it is conducive to appropriate interventions. Nevertheless, individuals may want to undergo genetic tests to determine their risk for Alzheimer's or other diseases even if there is no preventive treatment to date.[64] This situation shows that the concept of "clinical utility" may not apply to the particular preferences of individuals. Genetic tests may have a subjective value depending on their meaning for the particular life of an individual.[65] Beauchamp's and Childress' recommendation on this issue is helpful. They claim that "the subjective standard"[66] is the best criteria for the disclosure of information, i.e. the need for information can vary from individual to individual, which means that there is no prior standard and it would have to be identified on a case-by-case basis. Clinical judgement can make a huge contribution to case-by-case identification in both the process of information and decision-making.[67] However, other mechanisms such as the medical education and training of patients as well as the support of their health-care decisions are necessary and should be encouraged.[68] Therefore, it is important to realize

---

[63] S. D. Grosse, M. J. Khoury, "What is the clinical utility of genetic testing?", in: *Genetics in Medicine*, 8(7)/2006, p. 448-450, p. 448.

[64] See E. M. Bunnik et al., "Personal genome testing", p. 13 f.

[65] See "The potential value of genotypic information to individuals includes better understanding of their own prognosis, risk, or susceptibility to disease, or that of family members to disease, whether that knowledge affects clinical management decisions or not." (S. D. Grosse et al., "What is the clinical utility of genetic testing?", p. 449).

[66] T. L. Beauchamp et al., *Principles of Biomedical Ethics*, p. 123.

[67] Nuffield Council on Bioethics, *Pharmacogenetics,* p. 60 f.

[68] See HHS, *Personalized Health Care*, p. 51.

that individuals need the support of others, especially clinicians, in order to obtain the appropriate information and understand it. Online medicine and genetic tests alone do not suffice.

There is no doubt that Personalized Medicine supports a nontraditional understanding of the relationship between physicians and patients. As already mentioned, the benefits and harms of Personalized Medicine to the autonomy of individuals are related to its "consumerist" understanding of the relationship between individuals and health-care providers. However, we should also recognize that this situation is not unique to Personalized Medicine. In medical health services, the strong focus on consumers is an old phenomenon. But if we want to improve the ethical benefits of Personalized Medicine with regard to autonomy, it is indisputable that ethical principles of business ethics should be introduced. This means that not only do consumers have to take responsibility for their own health-care decisions, but the health providers also have to guarantee the quality and accuracy of their direct-to-consumer services. Individuals as consumers must also be legally protected from fraud and have the right to a competent customer advisory service. Even online resources such as websites with information on medical health care or diseases can be improved through a system of accreditation. It has been correctly stated that "the success of Personalized Medicine depends on having accurate diagnostic tests that identify patients who can benefit from targeted therapies."[69] Only if information tools are accurate and reliable, i.e. free from empty promises, lies and false advertising, can an individual's autonomy really be respected and not used as an object of manipulation.

---

[69] M. A. Hamburg et al., "The Path to Personalized Medicine", p. 2.

Personalized Healthcare: Focus on Individuality

Harald MATERN

Abstract: Ethical analyses of the implications of "personalized" or "individualized" healthcare state a gap between patients' expectations and the offering which is actually supplied under this name. When developing a vision for future research and therapy, this gap should be taken seriously. In this study several constituent moments of what in the modern philosophical and theological debate is called "personality" or "individuality" are presented. The discussion of these concepts is meant as heuristics for both: further social research in order to take into account the self-understanding of modern individuals and, in a rather meta-ethical perspective, the question to what extent the positions presented can claim ethical relevance in this special case.

1 Introduction

"Personalized" or "Individualized Healthcare" is the name of both a trend in medical research and a vision of healthcare systems focused on "personal" or "individual" needs and concerns in such different areas as diagnosis, prognosis and therapy, especially with respect to diseases of a more complex manner.[1] Regarding medical research, current interests tend to biomarker-based stratification whilst models of "individualized" medication and therapy[2], including personalized prosthetics on the one hand, the hope for a better collaboration with patients concerning their behavior with respect to diets, the consummation of drugs and the importance of physi-

---

[1] This definition is anything but clear. See P. Dabrock: "Die konstruierte Realität der sog. Individualisierten Medizin. Sozialethische und theologische Anmerkungen.", in: V. Schumpelick, B. Vogel (Eds.), *Medizin nach Maß. Individualisierte Medizin – Wunsch und Wirklichkeit*, Freiburg/Basel/Wien 2011, p. 239-267, p. 240.

[2] Individual differences concerning the susceptibility to different diseases are to be taken into account here, see J. M. Meyer, G. S. Ginsburg, "The path to Personalized Medicine", in: *Current Opinion in Chemical Biology*, 6(4)/2002, p. 434–438.

cal activities on the other hand[3], are understood as to belong to the area of "Personalized Healthcare".[4]

There are, as I believe, two main points to be stressed here when we deliberate ethical concerns raised by or linked to these new developments. The first observation to be made is that there is a gap between the expectations of individuals receiving medical treatment and the character of treatment offered under the title of "personalized" or "individualized" healthcare.[5] So

---

[3] See also the "typology" presented in B. Hüsing, J. Hartig, B. Bührlen, T. Reiß, S. Gaisser (Eds.), *Individualisierte Medizin und Gesundheitssystem*, TAB-Arbeitsbericht 126, Berlin 2008, p. 11, 129 ff., which distinguishes five types of individualization being relied on in current Personalized Healthcare research and therapy development. These are outlined as follows: "Zu den Faktoren, die die Entstehung und den Verlauf von Krankheiten beeinflussen, zählen verschiedene Umweltfaktoren und -einflüsse, Lebensführung und Lebensstil, Ernährung, genetische Faktoren und Unterschiede in der Genexpression und -regulation, psychische Faktoren sowie der Sozialstatus mit dem damit verbundenen sozialen Umfeld und den sozial geprägten Kompetenzen. Auch Alter, Geschlecht und Rasse sind relevant.", (B. Hüsing et al., *Individualisierte Medizin und Gesundheitssystem*, p. 39). See also the typology presented in: Nuffield Council on Bioethics (Eds.), *Medical profiling and online medicine: the ethics of 'personalised healthcare' in a consumer age*, London 2010, p. 30.

[4] See W. Niederlag, H. U. Lemke, O. Rienhoff, "Personalisierte Medizin und individuelle Gesundheitsversorgung. Medizin- und informationstechnische Aspekte.", in: *Bundesgesundheitsblatt*, 53(8)/2010, p. 776-782, p. 776.

[5] See P. Dabrock, "Die konstruierte Realität", p. 255 ff.; B. Hüsing et al., *Individualisierte Medizin und Gesundheitssystem*, p. 22, p. 44. It is, first of all, the "psychic" dimension, which is of importance here. In this analysis, I will consider this fact as pointing to the shape and content of the patients' self-awareness and as well their relationship to the medical and/or healthcare systems. Furthermore, the creation of an infrastructure of psycho-social caretaking seems to be essential when developing "individualized" healthcare systems. The same applies for psycho-social support concerning the handling of diseases. See G. Marstedt, S. Moebus (Eds.), *Inanspruchnahme alternativer Methoden in der Medizin. Gesundheitsberichterstattung des Bundes*, Berlin 2002, p. 22 f. and B. Hüsing et al., *Individualisierte Medizin und Gesundheitssystem*, p. 247. Concerning the concept of individuality which regards persons "as a whole", see: Nuffield Council on Bioethics, *Medical profiling and online medicine*, p. 30. At the same time, the question of the patient autonomy regarding the decision-making in therapeutical contexts should be discussed (which I will not do as extensively as could be necessary). See the analyses by D. Klemperer, "Shared Decision Making und Patientenzentrierung – vom Paternalismus zur Partnerschaft in der Medizin. Teil 1: Modelle der Arzt-Patient-Beziehung", in: *Balint Journal*, 6/2005b, p. 71-79; D. Klemperer, "Shared Decision Making und Patientenzentrierung – vom Paternalismus zur Partnerschaft in der Medizin. Teil 2: Risikokommunikation, Interessenkonflikte, Effekte von Patienten-

the question to be raised at first will point to our understanding of "individuality" in order to comprehend more clearly what we are talking about when we question the different concepts of individuality implicit in the patients' expectations and the treatment offered. The second point I shall like to highlight is the profound uncertainty or at least ambiguity concerning the concept of individuality itself when dealt with in ethical contexts. Combining these two points I will shift the focus on the concept of "individuality" in the modern (social) philosophical and theological discourse. This does not implicate that we take these traditions as normative for what individuality should "be" or should be taken as; but rather that they will be used in a heuristic approach that ascribes to the belief that philosophy and/or theology themselves are attempts to stress topics of individual and social concern and reformulate them in an analytical and rationalized manner. "Individuality" thus is perceived as a frame which impregnates modern concepts of the hermeneutics of self.

Before we can focus on individuality there is one more observation to be made. In many cases, "person" and "individual" are, at least in the German language, used almost synonymously. The tradition we are going to follow below makes a distinction between personality and individuality – and it is that difference which will grow important because of the ethical implications of its meaning. In the German-speaking tradition, the individual is, semantically spoken, 'more' than a person. It is a distinct, specific person. Many of the implications of this terminological distinction are, as far as I understand, not to be found in the English-speaking world, or, rather the semantic overlaps of 'individuality' as compared to "personality' are already comprised in the term 'personality' in the English language[6]. I will analyze this question further in Chapter 1.1. This means that focusing on Personalized Healthcare or Individualized Medicine has similar implications concerning the hermeneutics of self. And these implications are the main issues in what later on is to become an ethical discussion of a current

---

beteiligung", in: *Balint Journal*, 6(4)/2005a, p. 115–123.

[6] See the synonymous use of "person" and "individual" in Nuffield Council on Bioethics, *Medical profiling and online medicine*, p. 51 (here, individuality is very closely linked to "personal autonomy", a concept which does nevertheless not comprehend all material aspects of individuality as pointed out below. Furthermore, it is not clear at all where the basic values this report relies on (see Chapter 3) are derived from).

trend in medical research and therapeutic practice.

In what follows, "individuality" is to be understood as a manner of self-description and self-understanding underlying or shaping the "normal" way modern individuals tend to understand and express themselves. This "subjective" aspect of what can be called a "hermeneutical" approach corresponds to a "collective" one: In modern, complex societies, it is having passed through a process of functional differentiation, where a concept of "individuality" in its vast and profound meaning as pointed out below makes sense. "Individuality" is, as we will see, a concept implicit in the reflexive self-description of modern societies, stressing their internal complexity (and with it individuality) as an internalized opposition resulting from self-observation.

I will, in a second step, point out eight aspects or moments which are supposed to necessarily belong to the view we do have on what should be called "individuality" – and which is, of course, as "real" as any concept implicit in our cultural and moral practices (such as "freedom", "values" etc). They are discursive realities, but nevertheless, they become practical realities as they are relied on within the processes of our decision-making and acting.[7]

Finally, I will further the thesis that taking into account the variety of moments implicit in our self-understanding as individuals (including symbols of "metaphysical" entities or relationships such as "soul", "freedom" and "belief", the discursive realities mentioned earlier) will not only shed light on the popular image of what is called "Personalized Healthcare" or "Individualized Medicine" but close the gap between the patients' expectations and the treatment available (which, incidentally, will strengthen the confidential relationship between patients and medics). I will at least raise the question if doing so could not perhaps improve the diagnostical, prognostical and therapeutic efficiency of personalized treatments as well. This idea has already been stressed. There are demands to take psychosocial and environmental influences on the patients' reality into account when trying to evolve "individualized" or personalized therapeutical and diagnostical concepts.[8] I will champion the thesis that this does not only

---

[7]   This understanding of "reality" is, of course, close to the Kantian approach.

[8]   B. Hüsing et al., *Individualisierte Medizin und Gesundheitssystem*, p. 27, 297. See the table presented in Nuffield Council on Bioethics, *Medical profiling and online medicine,*

require qualitative studies from a societal study perspective[9], but that a systematic analysis of what it is we call "individuality" will affect the shape of such studies. Religion, as will be claimed below, plays a fundamental role in the integration of the moments of individuality to be described.

1.1 Systematic perspectives

Before diving deeper into the conceptual structure of our self-understanding as individuals, I will mention some conceptual differentiations in order to sharpen the tools for our analysis.

Individualization and Individualism

When sociologists talk about "individualization", they are usually addressing a process or evolution going along with the increasing complexity and internal (functional) differentiation of modern societies. The term "individualization" in this context is to be understood as a description of the increasing importance of the habits, potentials and acts of individual persons in functional relation to their societal environment.[10] This is a rather formal description of what "individualization" can mean.

We can identify another kind of use of this term with a more material meaning. Social diagnostics-related and ethically oriented texts tend to stress this part of the semantics of "individualization". In this context it denotes the imperatives of "risky freedom"[11], addressing the single person within modern societies, forcing the individual to individualize his or her

---

p. 183.

[9] B. Hüsing et al., *Individualisierte Medizin und Gesundheitssystem*, p. 300.

[10] For an overview of different types of concepts of individualization and individuality within sociological research and theory see M. Schroer (Ed.), *Das Individuum der Gesellschaft. Synchrone und diachrone Theorieperspektiven*, Frankfurt a. M. 2001. For a common perspective see as well H. Lübbe, "Gleichheit macht frei. Warum die sogenannte Massengesellschaft Individualisierungsprozesse begünstigt", in: V. Schumpelick, B. Vogel (Eds.), *Medizin nach Maß. Individualisierte Medizin – Wunsch und Wirklichkeit*, Freiburg/Basel/Wien 2011, p. 411-438.

[11] See U. Beck, E. Beck-Gernsheim, "Individualisierung in modernen Gesellschaften – Perspektiven und Kontroversen einer subjektorientierten Soziologie", in: U. Beck; E. Beck-Gernsheim (Eds.), *Riskante Freiheiten. Individualisierung in modernen Gesellschaften*, Frankfurt a.M. 1994, p. 10-39, p. 18.

manners and behavior. "Individualization" as a result becomes a moralized term to be applied in a manner critical of societal structures and institutions. In this sense, "individualization" is addressed explicitly as a part of people's self-understanding with a huge impact on their decisions and actions as well as their psychological stability. In a more 'active' sense, this meaning of individualization points to "individualism" as a form of self-understanding and behavior internalized in the persons who constitute modern societies.[12]

Individuality

The concept of "individuality" can also be understood in a more formal and material sense. In a formal perspective, "individuality" is an attribute of an entity which turns out to be qualitatively different from another entity in at least one aspect (*principium individuationis*). Turning to its material sense, "individuality" focuses on the relevance this difference from others has *for* the individual *themselves*. When applied in this sense, "individuality" ends up denoting "character" or "personal style". This aspect, along with the material meaning of "individualization", will become of greater importance for the present analysis.

Individuality, Personality, Subjectivity[13]

Apart from the different meanings "individuality" can acquire when used in a more formal or material sense, there is a certain ambiguity inherent in the

---

12 See N. Luhmann, "Individuum, Individualität, Individualismus", in: N. Luhmann (Ed.), *Gesellschaftsstruktur und Semantik. Studien zur Wissenssoziologie der modernen Gesellschaft Bd. 3*, Frankfurt a. M. 1993, p. 149-258. For a rather critical approach see the collected essays in: C. Taylor (Ed.), *Negative Freiheit? Zur Kritik des neuzeitlichen Individualismus*, Frankfurt a. M. 1992; C. Taylor (Ed.), *Das Unbehagen an der Moderne*, Frankfurt a. M. 1995.
13 See M. Frank (Ed.), *Die Unhintergehbarkeit von Individualität. Reflexionen über Subjekt, Person und Individuum aus Anlaß ihrer 'postmodernen' Toterklärung*, Frankfurt a. M. 1986. For an analytic approach see also M. Quante (Ed.), *Person*, Berlin 2007. Quante distinguishes between a rather normative, qualitative and a sortal meaning of the term "person". His approach on personal individuality is based on individual biographies (see p. 158 ff.) and thus comprises several of the aspects of individuality which I mention in my enquiry.

term itself. This ambiguity was pointed out by the German social philosopher Georg Simmel whom I will follow in the distinctions he made.[14] Firstly, "individuality" can be used quasi-synonymously with "subjectivity" as the capability to carry out self-determined actions. Self-determination means independence with reference to agency going along with the *numeric* distinction of the agent's subjectivity while subjectivity is meant to be a capability common to all rational beings. This is the viewpoint stressed by Kant, and, analytically more profound, by J.G. Fichte. Secondly, "individuality" can mean *qualitative* difference of the individual from all other individuals. This aspect of meaning was emphasized by Goethe and certain German Romanticists like Schleiermacher in his early works. Confusing both aspects semantically can lead to a lack of precision when dealing with individuality.

Dabrock[15] points out that the problem with the terminology used in the promotion of Personalized Healthcare deals rather with "personality" than with "individuality". It is true that some of the aspects or moments of individuality mentioned below are strongly related to the personality-bound tradition in Christian theology (especially those concerning communicational relations, below summarized under the topic of "intersubjectivity"). What I am trying to stress is, nevertheless, another perspective on the problem. While "personality", at least in the German-speaking tradition, points more or less exclusively to intersubjectively constituted relationships and thus communication, the problem of "individuality", is linked more strongly with matters of self-consciousness. Communicational processes appear, in this perspective, as a constitutive moment or aspect of self-awareness or a concept of self. Furthermore, "individuality" is "more" than "personality". Individuality cannot be defined. While "personality" is a commonly

---

[14] See G. Simmel, "Der Individualismus der modernen Zeit", in: G. Simmel (Ed.), *Individualismus der modernen Zeit und andere soziologische Abhandlungen*, Frankfurt a. M. 2008, p. 346-354. See also: G. Simmel, "Die Großstädte und das Geistesleben", in: G. Simmel (Ed.), *Individualismus der modernen Zeit und andere soziologische Abhandlungen*, Frankfurt a. M. 2008, p. 319-333. The ethical problems implicit in this ambiguity were analyzed by Simmel with reference to Kant and the ethical tradition following him in the essay "Das individuelle Gesetz", in: G. Simmel, *Das individuelle Gesetz. Philosophische Exkurse*. Edited by M. Landmann [1987], Frankfurt a. M. 1987, p. 174-230.

[15] P. Dabrock, "Die konstruierte Realität", p. 241.

applicable concept when dealing with human beings, "individuality", in the emphatic meaning employed below, is that specific personality which in the first term is only fully aware of *myself*. The communicational process of recognition is, logically speaking, secondary and only of relevance when mediated by *my* self-consciousness. When J. Heinrichs mentions four constitutive relations of personality (which are also mentioned below), it is firstly the ineffability by common concepts and secondly the "mediatedness" by the also ineffable individual self-consciousness, which lead me to focus on individuality and not on personality in this study. There is a third reason as well: When in the English-speaking tradition, the sense of "possession" is among the connotations of "personality"[16], I will claim that this sense is also comprised in the German "Individualität", which in the early 19th century Schleiermacher synonymously called "Eigenthümlichkeit".

Nevertheless, this choice of concept does neither mean that "personality" is of no importance here, nor that the problems concerning "personality" are of less importance to the ethical reflection concerning IM/PH. It is even true that the discussion about the specifications of "personality" is strongly linked to the debate about the importance of "individuality" in its historic extent. But the special emphasis on qualitative difference concerning individuality is peculiar to the discussion in European modernity, specifically the German Romanticism and its offshoots until today. What I want to stress then is that focusing on "individual" persons sharpens the problematic, extends and specifies it[17]. Additionally, the topic of "individuality" is of special relevance to the ethical reflections of the German-speaking tradition of modern protestant theology.

Individual(s)

The individual, of whom individuality is predicted, is, as could already be seen above, not sufficiently described if addressed merely as a unity in a logical sense.[18] In fact, it has to be characterized as the principle of identity of a complex unity in time and space. The individual, when applied as a

---

[16] See P. Dabrock, "Die konstruierte Realität", p. 241.

[17] When preferring the name "individualized" healthcare, one must admit that a really "individualized" medicine which would apply therapies to "individuals" in the emphatic sense, is practically out of reach. See P. Dabrock, "Die konstruierte Realität", p. 242.

[18] See N. Luhmann, "Individuum, Individualität, Individualismus", p. 194.

term in this formal sense, is figuratively speaking the description of the inversion of a multi-digit relation.

The "individual" in a more material sense of their meaning usually describes the self-referential and, for instance, self-conscious person being able to predicate "individuality" of themselves. The "individual" if addressed in this manner, means an individual subject.

1.2 Individuality as a parameter of description

Individuality, as already pointed out above, will be understood in this analysis as a constitutive parameter of the praxis of self-description in modern societies. This perspective does not only refer to collectives in a systemic manner. In fact, it addresses the self-understanding of individual persons as well. As a matter of fact, I will not be questioning the ontological or metaphysical status of this self-reference.[19] What is taken to be crucial in this analysis is the practical importance and impact of such self-reference. What I am doing here is to attribute hermeneutical-practical significance to the semantic field of "individuality" etc. as described above.

Self-description of societies

Niklas Luhmann alluded that in the beginnings of the 18th century the discursive amalgamation of two concepts took place in Western Europe, which since then have been autonomously discussed. This amalgamation will be critical to our understanding of individuality as what Luhmann focused on is the now established semantical unification of the concepts of "individuality" and "subjectivity".[20] Individuality can thus be understood as a form of semantical augmentation of subjectivity. That means that subjectivity, i.e. the transcendental capability of freedom which forms the basis of any

---

[19] Luhmann, for instance, understands the "'institutionalization' of individualism" as a result of the reflexivity constitutive for modern "society itself". See N. Luhmann, "Individuum, Individualität, Individualismus", p. 151. Luhmann thus understands "society" as the subject of individualization. Be this true or not, it would not challenge the view presented in this analysis, namely that 'individuality' is the shape and content of modern individuals' self-awareness which has, indeed, practical implications and hence a cultural-pragmatic 'reality' of its own.

[20] See N. Luhmann, "Individuum, Individualität, Individualismus", p. 208.

concept of morality relying on autonomy, is being augmented in a reflexive manner, now pointing to the concrete individual instead of the subjectivity which is, as a capability, general amongst rational beings.

However, it must be observed that mere reflexivity (in the meaning of self-reference *and* self-determination) is not sufficient in order to characterize the self-description of modern individuals.[21] Individuality is the symbol of a multi-digit relation.

Self-description of individual persons

The self-referring[22] individual is the "other" of society. But being this, they are understood in another kind of oppositional relation: one person amongst plural others. They are even more than that: the principles of their constitution form a deficient concept. "Individuum est ineffabile", Goethe wrote to J. C. Lavater when asked for the principles of his understanding of the possibilities of conceptually focusing mankind.[23] It is, on the one hand, one of the characteristic aspects of individuals that they cannot possibly

---

[21] Luhmann was challenged by different scholars reproofing his relying only on reflexivity as constituent principle of individual self-awareness as reductionist. See M. Frank (Ed.), *Selbstbewusstsein und Selbsterkenntnis. Essays zur analytischen Philosophie der Subjektivität*, Stuttgart 1991, p. 72; U. Barth, "Der ethische Individualitätsgedanke beim frühen Schleiermacher", in: G. Jerouschek, A. Sames (Eds.), *Aufklärung und Erneuerung. Beiträge zur Geschichte der Universität Halle im ersten Jahrhundert ihres Bestehens (1694-1806)*, Hanau/Halle 1994, p. 309-331, p. 311. I will hold this view in my analysis as far as it concerns the individuals' self-awareness.

[22] There is an ambiguity in the term "reflexivity". It can mean both: pre-rational self-reference or self-awareness and rational, language-bound self-reference which implies, through semiotical ostentation, a certain objectivization of one-self. While we believe of the capability of self-awareness that it owes to some classes of non-human beings (many species of 'animals') as well, reflexivity in the second sense is exclusive to rational beings capable of language. This sense of the term is implied as well when dealing with self-determination. The prevalence of one or the other sense of the word when dealing with self-consciousness is a topic of philosophical debate.

[23] So Goethe in a letter to Johann Casper Lavater, September 20th, 1780 (Weimarer Ausgabe, edited by P. Raabe, Band IV, 4, ND München 1987, p. 300). For its poetic context, see: F. Jannidis, "'Individuum est ineffabile'. Zur Veränderung der Individualitätssemantik im 18. Jahrhundert und ihrer Auswirkung auf die Figurenkonzeption im Roman", in: *Aufklärung*, 9(2)/1996, p. 77-110. The concept of individuality as undeterminable itself is ancient. My quoting it here is owed to the special shape and importance it grew to become in Western Europe modernity.

be determined as a mere example of a concept. Turning to the possibilities of addressing individuality (being taken into account as the shape of self-description of modern [collective] subjects), this means that the discourse about individuality must veil this impossibility in order to grant the possibility of communication and action itself by suggesting determinateness. It does so by – regarding its form – becoming symbolic.

On the other hand, this implies that "individuality" shapes the action-guiding views of any subject, and hence their cultural pragmatics. As such, "individuality" is not only the shape but becomes part of the content of symbolic self-predications of modern subjects. It is this last perspective which will be of some importance to us when we turn to analyze the ethical implications of the above mentioned gap between patients' expectations and "objectivized" individuality as laid down implicitly within the offers of Personalized Healthcare, which we chose as a starting point for our analysis.

In what follows, I will now turn to point out eight aspects of our symbolic concept of individuality as laid down in rationalized form in philosophical and theological analyses. It is of considerable importance that especially those approaches with a certain rooting in theology or at least philosophy of religion have contributed a lot in the conceptualization of the symbolic material[24] – a conceptualization which renders the task of describing "moments of individuality" easier to us now.

---

[24] The history of modern (German speaking) protestant theology can be read as a reflection on increasing societal and psychological processes of individualization (all meanings mentioned above are implied here). See G. Pfleiderer, "Protestantische Individualitätsreligion?", in: W. Gräb, L. Charbonnier (Eds.), *Individualität. Genese und Konzeption einer Leitkategorie humaner Selbstdeutung*, Berlin 2012, p. 372-404. As an addition to the scholars mentioned by Pfleiderer one could for example stress the ethics of Wilhelm Herrmann as a perfect example of the impact individualist concepts have had on theological and philosophical reflections of German scholars.

Due to this fact, the question arises, in which extension, if any, the protestant religion contributed to the shaping of the modern western-European societies. We will not discuss this topic in this place. As an example I refer to Ernst Troeltsch, whose reflections on the linkage between religion and modernity are basically shaped by the concept of individuality. See A. Heit, "Alt- und Neuprotestantismus bei Ernst Troeltsch", in: A. Heit., G. Pfleiderer (Eds.), *Protestantisches Ethos und moderne Kultur*, Zürich 2008, p. 55-78, p. 77.

It is no accident that at the beginning of modernity, Hegel contributed to Luther's turn to the subjectivity of faith. See G. W. F. Hegel, *Vorlesungen über die Philosophie der Geschichte*, Edited by H. Glockner [1949], Berlin 1848, p. 499 f.

Nevertheless, it must stay clear that these "moments", although in the following they are presented in a somewhat systematic manner, are always moments of *specific* systematics. Depending on the importance one attributes to each of these moments, their relevance concerning the "whole" of individuality changes. We will return to this point in the final chapter.

2 Constituent moments of individuality

2.1 Freedom, autonomy, self-determination

One of the constituent moments of individuality which has a broad impact on today's ethical discussions, especially in the range of topics with a healthcare-ethics-background, is the question whether there is any such thing as transcendental freedom in rational (human) beings, which allows us to address them as potential moral subjects. This conception of freedom or subjectivity, underlying for instance all discourses about "informed consent" or "patients' autonomy" is, obviously, the Kantian one. It forms the basis for modern conceptions of individuality – but it is not the same idea. The idea of freedom stressed in the Kantian approach, when taken as a matter of fact, grants the rational being the potential of self-determination. This capability, i.e. the practical capability of determining one's own goals, is nevertheless in no way comparable to what we call individuality today. It is, in a certain manner, opposed to the complex concept of individuality, since intelligible freedom in the Kantian Tradition is what distinguishes rational beings from animals, as a class of entities of which any member first of all is an example, as a *general* capability which is *in all the same* (as reason is one and general – the guarantee for the possibility or the valor of logics, for example). Self-determination may in no way be confused with individuality[25] although the first is comprised in the second.

2.2 Identification and Identifying

Individuality results, in one perspective, from discursive ostentation: The individual shall be determinate and must be addressed as such both in a

---

[25] So does Gerhardt in: V. Gerhardt (Ed.), *Selbstbestimmung. Das Prinzip der Individualität*, Stuttgart 2007.

distinguishing and identifying manner. From the outside, identification will be reached through the demarcation of a temporal-spatial position which grants the coordinates for the individual's identity.[26] In the case of the individual being a person, reflexive self-identifying as an act is at least as important for the constitution of individuality as is the identification of "outside" objects as such or as persons (only persons can identify persons).[27]

The relation described can be inverted: It may be not the act of reflexive self-identifying but the internalized "view of the other" which individualizes me by identification.[28] Identification by others brings with it the danger of complete determination, which is a forced and objectifying type of individualization. This determination is indeed not restricted to discursive practices but may also involve the influence exercised by societal-political institutions and their scientific fostering by the humanities.[29] In a more formal description, when we hark back to the starting point that "individuality" is the symbol for a multi-digit relation, we will at this point only sharpen our attention for the insight that the stability of any relation is endangered by the transformation of a symmetrical structure into an asymmetrical one (or, if constituted yet as such, by asymmetry in general).[30]

---

[26] See P. F. Strawson (Ed.), *Individuals*, London 1959, p. 23 ff.

[27] Strawson, *Individuals*, p. 131. The individual's self-identifying presupposes its identity. This is to consider as well when dealing with biography. This presupposition of identity (which is also the basis of what we have called "autonomy") is being tackled in "postmodern" approaches, at least if concerned as substantial. I will argue, that, whether or not there "is" (in a substantial sense) anything like, for example an "I" as an identical ground for the aspects mentioned, we must at least admit that this identity is a concept that we have to admit as a practical reality. (Even when talking of fragmentation we need a point of identity to refer to in order to measure the degree of fragmentation – in comparison to something that was or would be whole).

[28] Nevertheless, the "view of the other" as internalized, is mediated by an act of consciousness.

[29] We will come back to this point in the final chapter. For the moment, see M. Foucault, "Das Subjekt und die Macht", in: H. L. Dreyfus, P. Rabinow (Eds.), *Michel Foucault. Jenseits von Strukturalismus und Hermeneutik*, Frankfurt a. M. 1987, p. 243-261; for the genealogy of modern concepts of self and individuality see M. Foucault, "Technologien des Selbst", in: M. Foucault, R. Martin, L. H. Martin, W. E. Paden, K. S.Rothwell, H. Gutman, P. H. Hutton (Eds.), *Technologien des Selbst*, Frankfurt a. M. 1993, p. 24-62. For critics and affirmation see T. Junge (Ed.), *Gouvernementalität der Wissensgesellschaft. Politik und Subjektivität unter dem Regime des Wissens*, Bielefeld 2008, p. 257-295 (especially chapter 8: "Der Hirte seiner selbst: Subjektivität und Politik").

2.3 Corporeity

What external identification as well as the internal act of self-identifying rely on is spatial and temporal continuity which means identity is maintained through temporal and spatial changes. The symbol or demarcation of this identity is, as objectivized, the body. When taking into account that reflexivity or the act of self-identifying is one of the constituent moments of individuality as the shape and content of self-understanding of persons, "body" does not sufficiently describe the perception we have of ourselves being that continuous entity.[31] Phenomenological philosophy thus introduced the term of "corporeity" in this discussion. In the interior perception of itself, the individual does not "have" a body but "is" corporal. The intelligible continuity of the "I" which goes along with any self-reference gets intertwined with the (formerly addressed as "outside") phenomenal continuity of the body in time and space.[32] Corporeity is an aesthetical or rather phenomenological concept which has a profound share on the description of individuality. It is, as such, symbol for the special form of identity individuals are.

The individual's corporeity as a phenomenological principle of identity refers to another constituent moment of individuality. The individual is corporal history. Biography is embodied memory which is essentially linked with the anticipation of future – in a corporal manner, as an intellectual and sensual perceptional anticipation including the presentation of future interaction.

We will first turn to the description of interaction before dealing with biography.

---

[30] We will return to this aspect later. For the impact of symmetry/asymmetry in relational concepts of individuality see J. Dierken, "Riskiertes Selbstsein. Individualität und ihre (religiösen) Deutungen", in: W. Gräb, L. Charbonnier (Eds.), *Individualität. Genese und Konzeption einer Leitkategorie humaner Selbstdeutung*, Berlin 2012, p. 329-347.

[31] Manfred Frank points out that the "body" is exactly not the entity we can rely on in order to grant individual identity. See M. Frank, *Selbstbewusstsein und Selbsterkenntnis*, p. 44.

[32] See B. Waldenfels (Ed.), *Das leibliche Selbst. Vorlesungen zur Phänomenologie des Leibes*, Frankfurt a. M. 2000, p. 42.

2.4 Intersubjectivity and recognition

It is the interaction of individuals which reciprocally strengthens the boundaries of their corporeal identity. The historical roots of current theories of intersubjectivity and recognition have their roots in the early Fichtean philosophy of mind. J.G. Fichte, the most famous Kantian of his era, projected since the very beginnings of his career the transformation of the Kantian distinction between transcendental and empirical subjectivity. As a result, Fichte developed his early philosophy of "I", which constituted its boundaries in relation to its intelligible opposition, the Non-I.[33] In the following years, Fichte extended his theory in order for it to be capable of comprehending "real" interaction, nevertheless from a merely intelligible point of view. It should not only be the Non-I as determinate opposition of the I but another I which was meant to constitute the individuality of the I.[34] The outcome of the early Fichtean project was the embedding of Kantian subjectivity in a theory of (intelligible) interaction and reciprocal recognition: a relational theory of individual subjectivity was born, which had a broad impact on modern social philosophy.[35]

In current discussions on intersubjectivity and recognition we find the extension of what Fichte discussed on a purely intellectual level into a "realistic" point of view. Jürgen Habermas, for instance, understands individuality relying strongly on the model of communicational interaction developed by G.H. Mead, namely as a result of intersubjective communication comprehended as a form of "action" sui generis.[36] The social philosopher

---

[33] See J. G. Fichte, *Grundlage der gesamten Wissenschaftslehre als Handschrift für seine Zuhörer*. Edited by W. G. Jacobs [1997], Leipzig 1794, above all § 3. See as well D. Henrichs (Ed.), *Selbstverhältnisse. Gedanken und Auslegungen zu den Grundlagen der klassischen deutschen Philosophie*, Stuttgart 1982, p. 57-82.

[34] See J. G. Fichte, *Das System der Sittenlehre nach den Prinzipien der Wissenschaftslehre*. Edited by H. Verweyen [1995], Hamburg 1798, above all § 18: "Systematische Aufstellung der Bedingungen der Ichheit in ihrer Beziehung auf den Trieb nach absoluter Selbständigkeit".

[35] It is not my intention to establish a direct linkage between Fichte and modern social philosophy. But I hold the view that in Fichtes early philosophy the shape of what would become modern philosophy of intersubjectivity and recognition was shaped in a paradigmatical way.

[36] See J. Habermas, "Individuierung durch Vergesellschaftung. Zu George Herbert Meads Theorie der Subjektivität", in: J. Habermas (Ed.), *Nachmetaphysisches Denken*.

and ethicist Axel Honneth relies on Hegel (who in turn relied strongly on Fichte) in order to voice his theory of recognition with a (transcendentally grounded) pragmatic scope.[37]

The importance of intersubjective interaction and recognition for the shaping of the boundaries of individuals' identities notwithstanding, intersubjectivity and the mutual taking over of perspectives (which means, the appresentation of the other within my concept of me as an individual) as such are not sufficient for the description of what we call individuality. [38]

2.5 Self-presentation or "Expressivism" as a moment of self-constitution

The intelligible, communication-bound or pragmatic theories of intersubjectivity and recognition can be broadened in an aesthetical-pragmatical manner. The shape of this extension was formed in the early 19th century by the philosopher and theologian Friedrich D.E. Schleiermacher as a response to the Fichtean approach on the transformation of the Kantian theory of subjectivity. The individual should not only be self-conscientious and self-determining, they should not only be aware of the social frame of their self-consciousness, but they must express this awareness in such a symbolic manner which should comprehend both: self-awareness and awareness of the other.[39] In his later lectures on Christian Ethics, Schleiermacher highlights this "Darstellung", i.e. self-presentation which means "an activity

---

Philosophische Aufsätze, Frankfurt a. M. 1992, p. 187-241, p. 209.

[37] See A. Honneth (Ed.), *Leiden an Unbestimmtheit. Eine Reaktualisierung der Hegelschen Rechtsphilosophie*, Stuttgart 2001, p. 79-101.

[38] This point was averred by M. Frank (Ed.), *Selbstbewusstsein und Selbsterkenntnis,* p. 410-477, see also p. 410-416; for the hermeneutical or rather interpretationist implications of individuality as laid down in this analysis, see. p. 474-477.

[39] This concept already shaped form and content of Schleiermachers "Monologen" (F. D. E. Schleiermacher, *Monologen nebst den Vorarbeiten*. Edited by F. M. Schiele, H. Mulert [1978], Hamburg 1800). See also U. Barth, "Der ethische Individualitätsgedanke beim frühen Schleiermacher". Later on, the expressivist paradigm was adopted by Georg Simmel, see for example G. Simmel, "Die Großstädte und das Geistesleben", p. 328 f., where he states that a "Mensch nicht zu Ende ist mit den Grenzen seines Körpers oder des Bezirks, den er mit seiner Thätigkeit unmittelbar erfüllt, sondern erst mit der Summe der Wirkungen, die sich von ihm aus zeitlich und räumlich erstrecken" [that a human being is not wholly comprised within the limits of his body or the area which he immediately covers with his actions, but concludes only with the sum of effects which

through which man does not want to reach any [determined] goal"[40], but which nevertheless belongs to his individuality in a constitutive manner. Individuality in the full sense of the term is not constituted unless man expresses "the consciousness of his own being as absolutely completed"[41] – this consciousness is, by the way, in Schleiermacher's opinion only constituted in what he calls "religion" or "piety" (We will come back to that point later).

Due to the paradigm of expressivism or self-presentation, a material dimension is added to the theory of intersubjectivity and recognition as constituting moments of individuality.[42] Thus, individuality as shape and

---

sprawl from him in temporal and spatial extension, HM].

[40] F. D. E. Schleiermacher, *Die christliche Sitte nach den Grundsätzen der ev. Kirche im Zusammenhang dargestellt.* Edited by W. E. Müller [1999], [2]Berlin 1884, p. 37: "... [eine] Thätigkeit[], durch welche der Mensch nichts erreichen will" [English translation above by the author, HM]. This conception of "[self-]presenting action" was anticipated already in the early "Versuch einer Theorie des geselligen Betragens". In this text, society is presented under the form of an organism constituted in its liveliness by the "style" or "character" presented by anybody of its members. See F. D. E. Schleiermacher, "Versuch einer Theorie des geselligen Betragens", in: O. Braun, J. Bauer (Eds.), *Schleiermachers Werke*, Volume 2, Leipzig 1913, p. 3-31. In Schleiermacher's theology, the "[self-]presenting action" is the concept underlying his theory of service as its goal is described as presenting the "Bewußtsein der Seligkeit" [consciousness of blessedness] and, hence, the "total domination of the flesh by the spirit" ["Herrschaft des Geistes über das Fleisch", F. D. E. Schleiermacher, *Die christliche Sitte*, p. 527] in the medium of art. In his Philosophical Ethics, Schleiermacher described art as the language of religion by relying on the view that both in art and religion, it is the individuality of man which shapes the form of his communication (in difference to scientific communication which is shaped by general concepts. See: M. Moxter, "Zur Eigenart ästhetischer Erfahrung", in: E. Gräb-Schmidt, R. Preul (Eds.), *Ästhetik*, Marburger JahrbuchTheologie XXII, Leipzig 2010, p. 53-78, p. 60-64. "[Self-]presenting action" in Schleiermacher's theory is not in the first place a form of communication but it is in itself the completion of individuality – which means that the individuals' "status before the [self-]presentation is less complete than afterwards" (dass sein "Zustand vor der Darstellung ein unvollkommenerer ist, als nach der Darstellung",F. D. E. Schleiermacher, *Die christliche Sitte*, p. 37).

[41] "...das Bewußtsein des eigenen Seins als eines völlig abgeschlossenen", F. D. E. Schleiermacher, *Die christliche Sitte*, p. 36.

[42] B. W. Sockness has established an interesting linkage between the early roots of the Schleiermacherian theory of "Darstellung" and Charles Taylors' expressivist conception of the constitution of what he calls "self", see B. W. Sockness, "Schleiermacher and the ethics of authenticity. The Monologen of 1800", in: *Journal of Religious Ethics*,

content of self-hermeneutics or self-understanding is not only in a pragmatical but in an aesthetical manner subject to intersubjective hermeneutics as well. It is not only the practical boundaries of interaction but the unreachable nature of the other in conceptional terms[43], what constitutes a manner of hermeneutical interaction as a further constitutent moment of individuality. Recognition then must be restrained to a plurality of interpretations but cannot alone be the determining factor of individuality.

2.6 Determination by the Undeterminable: Religion as a moment of self-understanding

In order to constitute a consciousness of the wholeness of their own identity, the individual must, at least in one point, be determined. The determining factor cannot be the other as conceived as "nature", or corporeity, as corporeity is subject to changes through space and time (hence it can neither be the Kantian intelligible "I" which is, as a matter of fact, a general, not an individual attribute); it also cannot be the other individual, as the result of hermeneutical interaction will be plural and open to changes, as we have seen.

It is again the achievement of Friedrich Schleiermacher to have laid down a formal description of what one can call the religious dimension of self-awareness. The formality of his description is of great use to any non-foundationalist approach concerning the ethical implications of our hermeneutics of individuality. Following Schleiermacher, religion is that

---

32(3)/2004, p. 477–517.

[43] Concerning the "psychological" part of his hermeneutics (here with reference to the individuality of style, which in his conception is closely linked to the psychological individuality of the author), Schleiermacher promoted the combination of two methods, comparison and immediate visualization ["Anschauung"]. While comparison deals with common concepts and tries to subordinate the individual under one of these, the immediate visualization, although perceiving the whole of the other, lacks of communicability. Schleiermacher concludes: "Die unmittel[bare] Anschauung kommt nicht zur Mitteilbarkeit; die Vergleichung kommt nie zur wahren Individualität. Man muß beide miteinander vereinigen durch die Beziehung auf die Totalität des Möglichen." What follows from this is: "Die Eigentümlichkeit als Einheit nicht wiederzugeben; es bleibt immer etwas nicht zu Beschreibendes darin". (F. D. E. Schleiermacher, *Hermeneutik und Kritik*. Edited by M. Frank [1977], Berlin 1838, p. 119f.)

dimension of individuality which grants a principle of identity to the corporal and social dimension of self-awareness.[44] This principle takes over the systematic function of what is called "freedom" in the Kantian tradition. To Schleiermacher, this principle is appresented by the individual as the awareness of being determined by a "ground" which itself is not fully determinable.[45] This ground is indeterminable in a different sense to the other individual insofar it is not only the identical determining ground of me and the other but of the world as a whole.

Formulating a concept of religion in this merely formal manner provides the advantage of addressing a constituent principle of individuality as both infinite but not objective in a pre-critical sense of metaphysics. The material content of its symbolizations is, hence, to be understood as a result of individual interpretation – in a certain sense as an interpretation of individuality itself.

The precise form of the Schleiermacherian approach in conceptualizing religion enables or at least facilitates the communication between religious-bound reflections and non-religious discourses. It is, on the one hand, the hermeneutical approach to the conception of individuality (as explained with reference to intersubjectivity and recognition as well in 2.5) which

---

[44] See F. D. E. Schleiermacher, *Sämmtliche Werke. Dritte Abtheilung, Zur Philosophie 6. Psychologie.* Edited by L. George, Berlin 1862, p 211-213; E. Herms (Ed.), *Menschsein im Werden. Studien zu Schleiermacher*, Tübingen 2003, p. 192 ff.

[45] See F. D. E. Schleiermacher, *Sämmtliche Werke. Dritte Abtheilung, Zur Philosophie 4. 2. Dialektik.* Edited by L. Jonas, Berlin 1839, p. 150-152: "im Gefühl ist die im Denken und Wollen bloß vorausgesetzte absolute Einheit des idealen und realen wirklich vollzogen, da ist sie unmittelbares Bewusstsein, ursprünglich." [Within feeling, the absolute identity of the ideal and real is really consummated – which in thinking and willing was only relied on]. See also: U. Barth (Ed.), *Aufgeklärter Protestantismus*, Tübingen 2004, p. 353-385. Schleiermacher gives this philosophical conception a specific theological form, see: F. Scheiermacher, *Der christliche Glaube nach den Grundsätzen der Evangelischen Kirche im Zusammenhange dargestellt.* Edited by M. Redeker [1999], [7]Berlin 1830/31, p. 28. Schleiermacher calls this "awareness of absolute dependency" (Bewusstsein "schlechthinniger Abhängigkeit"). It is interesting that merely secular conceptions of autonomy and self-determination also take into account the reliance on at least one conceptionally indeterminable fact. Volker Gerhardt states, referring to "Selbstverwirklichung", that it relies on "the absolute in existence [Das Absolute im Dasein]" as an "original act, which we ourselves understand as unconditional [*ursprüngliche[r] Akt*, der von uns selbst als *bedingungslos* begriffen wird]", see V. Gerhard (Ed.), *Selbstbestimmung*, p. 414.

questions the mere facticity of self-awareness with regards to its ground or the different moments of its constitution. On the other hand, it is the reliance on a moment of indeterminacy within the logics of constitution of practical knowledge which renders this approach worthy of consideration in discussions fostering the ethical implications of the self-understanding of modern individuals in a merely secular perspective as well.

2.7 Biography

Biography is, in a certain manner, the counterpart of what above has been referred to as corporeity. Corporeity integrates the perception of both, spatial and temporal continuity of the individual. Analyzing intersubjectivity, expressivity and religion, we have conceived a possible principle of this identity. Biography is the manner in which individuals rely on such a principle in a more constructive way[46] in order to organize self-awareness as a historical view on temporarily and spatially seemingly disengaged facts in a sequential or rather narrative manner. Authorship of that self-narration is one of the integrating principles of individuality.[47] The organizational structure in combination with the integrated complex elements of one's biography is what renders it individual. The narrative form of its outcome points once more to the symbolic character of our expressions of individuality. They are, as already claimed above, open to interpretation, because it's only ourselves who can claim the authorship of symbolization – the generality of the principle relied on notwithstanding.

The "active" and practical (or better: constructive) connotations of the constitution of what we have called "biography" imply another moment of individuality we will have to take into account: "authorship" extends not only to the more resuming act of constituting and interpreting one's own

---

[46] The constructive character of biography, in a classic theory-of-action shape, is for example stressed by B. Geissler, M. Oechsle, "Lebensplanung als Konstruktion. Widersprüchliche Anforderungen aus Arbeitsmarkt und Familie und individuelle Lösungen im biographischen Handeln junger Frauen. Ergebnisse einer empirischen Studie.", in: U. Beck, E. Beck-Gernsheim (Eds.), *Riskante Freiheiten.Individualisierung in modernen Gesellschaften,* Frankfurt a. M. 1994, p.139-167, p. 139-144.

[47] For a current position, see J. Habermas, "Individuierung durch Vergesellschaftung", p. 191, 203.

biography *ex post* but to its practical shaping concerning our present and future.

2.8 Shaping of individuality

When I speak of the "shaping of individuality" I am referring to the practical influence we exercise on the development and shape of what we have described as "biography". This is the attempt to anticipate or imagine a vision which should serve it as a leading principle and, by doing so, transform its process into one which has a shape and goal of our own – "individual" – imprinting.[48] Others have used the term "handicraft-existence" ("Bastelexistenz") to describe this behavior which has in fact some critical implications, as it alludes to disintegrity and confusion. I will not hold this view on the shaping of individuality.

Nonetheless, there are at least two important points to be highlighted. First of all, the goal or guiding principle which man chooses to conceptualize his individuality. Secondly, but not less important, we have to consider the substance upon which the shaping is exercized. (Third, and a bit more complicated, we should not forget to ask who or what there is to exercise anything on anything not being identical with that anything to be shaped.) With the rise of genetical engineering and genome analysis, the individual perception of this given starting point for the act of shaping has been subjected to a fundamental transformation: The individual is often addressed as genetically determined – which could mean total transparency and openness to public concerning the principle of his individual identity. [49] If we

---

[48] Michel Foucault points out the fact that the ability of shaping one's own life is one of the constitutive characteristics of modern individuality. Thus, individuality is characterized by "die individualistische Einstellung, gekennzeichnet durch den absoluten Wert, den man dem Individuum in seiner Einzigkeit beilegt, und durch den Grad an Unabhängigkeit, der ihm gegenüber von der Gruppe, der es angehört, oder den Institutionen, denen es untersteht, zugestanden wird; die Hochschätzung des Privatlebens, das heißt das Ansehen, in dem die familiären Beziehungen, die Formen der häuslichen Aktivität und der Bereich der Erbinteressen stehen; endlich die Intensität der Selbstbeziehungen, das heißt der Formen, in denen man sich selbst zum Erkenntnisgegenstand und Handlungsbereich nehmen soll, um sich umzubilden, zu verbessern, zu läutern, sein Heil zu schaffen." M. Foucault (Ed.), *Die Sorge um sich*, Sexualität und Wahrheit 3, [10]Frankfurt a. M. 1989, p. 59.

[49] The discussion about "naked genes" can be understood as a result of this development.

take this determination for granted, most of the ideas mentioned above would lose their meaning.

Nevertheless, I will hold the view that what has been described as moments of individuality in the meaning of the self-understanding of modern man has a cultural-practical reality and impact which, for the moment, has not yet absorbed the idea of complete determination.[50] However, we cannot disregard the fact that the shaping of individuality has become a more or less public task.[51] This points once more to the ethical implications of the current concept of individuality as described above and the possible changes it will be subject to due to biopolitical shifts.

3 Ethical Implications

As I pointed out above, when dealing with ethical implications concerning concepts of individuality, it is not the conceptual "moments" alone which are of considerable importance but rather their complex unity and the systematics underlying their combination. Differences between concepts of individuality derive from the weight and systematic combination of the men-

See for the importance of publicity: H. Nowotny, G. Testa (Eds.), *Die gläsernen Gene. Die Erfindung des Individuums im molekularen Zeitalter*, Frankfurt a. M. 2009, p. 12-18, p. 70 ff.

[50] The idea of complete genetic determination – whether true or not – would not only destroy our concept of individuality but also the one of subjectivity in a moral sense as well. If we accepted that, we should rather go on and transform, for instance, our legal systems which depend upon the idea of individual responsibility which, in its case, relies fundamentally on the Kantian idea of autonomy.

It is rather misleading when Elisabeth Beck-Gernsheim points out: "Der moderne Mensch nimmt sein Schicksal selbst in die Hand. Er plant, er sieht vor, er kontrolliert und optimiert. Er folgt nicht mehr Gott und den Sternen. Die Gene sagen ihm jetzt, wie er sein Leben einrichten soll." (E. Beck- Gernsheim, "Gesundheit und Verantwortung im Zeitalter der Gentechnologie", in: E. Beck-Gernsheim, U. Beck (Eds.), *Riskante Freiheiten. Individualisierung in modernen Gesellschaften*, Frankfurt a. M., 1994, p. 316-335, p. 331) [Modern man takes matters into his own hands. He does no longer follow god and the stars. Genes tell him now how to live his life.] If the individuality were totally determined by genetic predisposition, there would not rest anybody to tell anything to about shaping his or her own life because the idea of autonomy would be a somewhat ridicule remark to a foreign epoch (not to mention the concept of individuality as described above).

[51] See H. Nowotny et al., *Die gläsernen Gene*, p. 136 f.

tioned moments. Individuality thus appears as a harmonic configuration of the elements mentioned. For example, communication-bound models concerning the constitution of individuality will stress the importance of dialogue. It is possible to highlight each of the moments implied. Following Fichte, one would champion the logical prevalence of the principle of identity (the "I") implicit in the individual's self-consciousness. The "other" with reference to whom I am constituted as an individual "me", appears first of all as limit or restriction of the "I". So, if any, there is an asymmetry or a logical decline from "I" to "me" to the "other". If one follows a rather Hegelian approach, the authority of the other counts more. It is not surprising that post-Hegelian approaches are able to estimate the "other" of "me" as logically primary. Asymmetries will be distinguished as a logical decline from "other" (or "the society") to "me".

Theological approaches will tend to champion the indeterminate moment of "God" as determining all other moments implied. Depending on whether one thinks this moment as mediated by the concrete "other" as appearing in communicational situations, or as primarily implicit in the individual self-consciousness, there will be other possibilities of asymmetrical configurations: "God" can appear as concrete "authority" of logical primacy, or rather as founding ground of the identity of consciousness which nevertheless is implicit in the construction of reality as mediated by self-consciousness.

These differences notwithstanding, what seems to be common to theological approaches (at least in the German-speaking modern protestant theology) is stressing the "intangibility" or transcendence of "God", be it in an ontological sense or a rather transcendental-philosophical meaning (in the so called "liberal" tradition). This is of some importance here: Christian theologians will stress the idea that within constitutional logics of individuality there will and must be at least one moment which in some way or other determines the whole process, while this moment itself can in no way be determined. The indeterminability of this moment is what grants not only individuality, but, as well, individual freedom, at least in a logical or rather meaning. Material or concrete freedom or rather the value of the individual as such will be derived from this logically primary moment of its constitution. Both points are strongly related with what we have called the "religious" moment of self-understanding – because it is this perspective which apparently grants a concept of self-determination and authorship of the own biography and life which relies on a principle outside the public sphere – outside in the same sense as it is outside of me, which was described above as a logical indetermination within the constitutional logic of individuality itself and as openness to the future.

The religious symbol for this reliance is the individual's relation to God. But in its secular conceptualization, this determined indeterminacy can be of some relevance for the individual.[52]

There are three points which I now want to mention as "ethical implications" of this analysis. They are strongly connected.

At first, we will have to strengthen the point that "Individualized Medicine" or "Personalized Healthcare" could be misunderstood. In the beginning of this analysis, we pointed out that this possible misunderstanding leads to the gap between patients' expectations on the one hand and the medical research being done or the possibilities of treatment being offered on the other hand.

What is called "personalization" or "individualization" of healthcare presents a very reduced view of individuality in comparison to the complex relational configuration of this manner of self-understanding of modern individuals as presented in part 2 of the analysis. "Individuality" would be reduced to be implicit "only" in the "body" – which turns out to be an "objectification" concerning the fact that corporeity as a form of being is one of the constituent moments of the appresentation of individuality in man's consciousness rather than having a body – and that even corporeity does not constitute the wholeness of what we call "individuality". This would imply an asymmetry which would consider the individual as constituted by a material aspect. It is clear that this cannot possibly be an implication of what

---

[52] The term of "Selbstverwirklichung" [self-realization] which is often used in similar contexts (see V. Gerhardt, *Selbstbestimmung*, p. 414 ff.), may go along with the self-understanding of some people. As a concept, it is rather cloudy as it relies on the metaphorics of ideal and realization or core and unfolding which would mean, philosophically speaking, that it substitutes the idea of "determination by the undeterminable" by "determined determination" or "determination by the determined", which leads to moral naturalism or determinism which is opposed to the concept of individuality presented in this analysis. This may be seen in an historical perspective as a modern continuation of the struggle between romanticists vs. the Philosophers of Enlightenment – in a systematic view it is the opposition of individuality and general subjectivity.

really "is" "personalized" or "individualized" healthcare. Thus it should be clear that the concept of "individuality" dealt with in the visions of "Individualized Medicine" is different from the one which is implicit in our reflections about our self-understanding. This difference should be marked terminologically as well.[53]

It could nevertheless be of great importance to the field of Personalized Healthcare to take into account not only the other moments of individuality mentioned above, but as well the "religious" side of it – be it in a formal or a more material way. Even if this had no impact on therapeutic efficiency, it would lead to the growth of confidence of patients about Personalized Healthcare and hence, help to close the "gap" observed in the relation between modern individuals and the medical and or the healthcare systems. That would mean to strengthen the psycho-social aspect of healthcare systems, the so-called "talking medicine", which is a desideratum surely not only from a theological point of view.

Secondly, returning to the starting point of our analysis, the patients' insecurity regarding Personalized Healthcare leads us straight to the question of intersubjectivity and recognition.[54] The "gap" pointed at stresses the relationship between patient and medic, between patient and the social public and, furthermore, between the patient and the institutionalized healthcare systems. It is thus a threat to the current conception of individuality, as it presents an asymmetrical relationship between objectifying identification from the 'outside' and the act of identifying oneself – with all the implications already mentioned.

This constitutes not only the point of departure of this analysis but also of such theories which claim the relation between the individual and an institutionalized "bio-power" to be critical.[55]

---

[53] "Stratification" seems to be a rather adequate name. See as well P. Dabrock, "Die konstruierte Realität", p. 243.

[54] This is the more "personality"-related ethical implication.

[55] See P. Gehring (Ed.), *Was ist Biomacht? Vom zweifelhaften Mehrwert des Lebens*, Frankfurt a. M. 2006, p. 55-74. This question is interesting when seen within in the context of the discussion on "rearing men", see P. Gehring, *Was ist Biomacht?*, p. 169-173, p. 182 f. See also: T. Lemke, "Die Regierung der Risiken. Von der Eugenik zur genetischen Gouvernementalität", in: U. Bröckling, S. Krasmann, T. Lemke (Eds.), *Gouvernementalität der Gegenwart. Studien zur Ökonomisierung des Sozialen*, Frankfurt a. M. 2000, p. 227-264. The concept of "bio-power" is different to that of "gouvernemental-

But there is a remarkable difference. Stressing asymmetry in this sense means that one really believes that "the society" or whatever concept is used in this place really *has* the power to determine individuality. Highlighting "bio-power" only works when power is *given* to what is considered "power" in such concepts and thus a concept of individuality is promoted, which from a theological standpoint could be called "reductionist". A Christian theological position would always stress the point, that even "power" must be considered to be derived from the principle of power which itself is transcendent to all material powers. This means, that there is, first of all, no reason to generally suspect "Personalized Healthcare" of threatening our individuality, but rather care for the design of its concrete proceedings.[56]

Thirdly, its theological scopus notwithstanding, this analysis in its main parts has been designed to provide not a norm but a *heuristics* of individuality. It has done so not by qualitative social research but by a systematical-historical approach to modern philosophy and theology. This is not meant to suggest its logical priority to social research but to give a framework to such analyses by providing a systematized overview of what individuality has been – and could possibly be nowadays – conceived as.

Thus, it will be necessary to strengthen the view that "individuality" as conceived in concepts of Individualized Medicine may in no case be used as a determining concept but must be applied in the sense of a heuristical-hermeneutical approach. If "individuality" in fact "was" what it is described to be in current concepts of Personalized Hpealthcare, there will not be, from a theological perspective, any need of calling it by that name.[57] What we can see further from more of a sociological perspective is that social differentiation brings with it semantic differentiations as well. What theolo-

---

ity", particularly in its more active meaning. In both cases, the focus is on the (political) terms of constitution of what we have called "individuality", as far as subjectivity and corporeity are seen together. In this meaning, one can talk about "bio-politics" as well, see G. Agamben (Ed.), *Homo sacer. Die Souveränität der Macht und das nackte Leben*, Frankfurt a. M. 2002, p. 127-162.

[56] So does P. Dabrock, "Die konstruierte Realität", p. 255-262.

[57] Even if one does not assume that the terminology used forms part of a marketing strategy, it is to admit that, "individualized" or "personalized" healthcare either must be considered a tautology (P. Dabrock, "Die konstruierte Realität", p. 239 f.) or is nothing but the result of a broader societal evolution towards differentiation and individualization (H. Lübbe, "Gleichheit macht frei", p. 427).

gians or philosophers call "individuality" and what, as we presumed in this analysis, coincides with the self-understanding of many people, is not necessarily the same as what is called "individuality" in the sphere of medicine and healthcare. This is a specific difficulty when dealing with the problem of special ethics. Nevertheless, as we have seen, there are reasons to believe that what we pointed out as constitutive for concepts of individuality from a philosophical and theological perspective may have its valence as well when applied to this special situation.

Further social research framed in the way above described should enlarge our knowledge about what individuality, if conceived as we did as a symbol for the multi-digit relationship in which modern individuals are constituted, really "is" – and which tasks this implies for a research- or therapy-bound program of Individualized Medicine.

Stratified Medicine: The Upholding of Eugenic Ideals?

Eugenics and Genetic Counseling

Reinhard HEIL

> "The judgment finds the facts that have been recited and that Carrie Buck 'is the probable potential parent of socially inadequate offspring, likewise afflicted, that she may be sexually sterilized without detriment to her general health and that her welfare and that of society will be promoted by her sterilization,' and thereupon makes the order. [...] Three generations of imbeciles are enough."
> U.S. Supreme Court, BUCK v. BELL, 274 U.S. 200 (1927)

> "It is ethically imperative that when genetic testing that may have significant implications for a person's health is being considered, genetic counselling should be made available in an appropriate manner. Genetic counselling should be non-directive, culturally adapted and consistent with the best interest of the person concerned."
> International Declaration on Human Genetic Data, Article 11 – Genetic Counselling

Abstract: The article addresses the question of whether genetic counseling is eugenic. The first part of the paper reconstructs the basic ideas of eugenics by reference to prominent eugenic positions (Francis Galton, Charles Davenport). Here, the paper considers that the idea of eugenics is not dependent on a particular scientific and political theory, but thrives in many different social climates. The second part of the paper gives a brief overview of different genetic counseling processes. The result is that there is no clear answer to the question of whether genetic counseling is eugenic or not. Genetic counseling is not inherently eugenic, but it can be used within a eugenic articulation in order to enforce eugenic goals. It is therefore always in danger of becoming eugenic.

1 Introduction

Genetic Counseling is one of the few procedures of the so-called Individ-ualized or Stratified Medicine which are already applied today. However, not only genetic counseling but "New Genetics" in general,[1,2] which try to establish relationships between genetic alterations and diseases and even traits of character by analyzing the genomes of larger and larger populations are suspicious of supporting old eugenic ideals. In this context it is talked about backdoor eugenics[3] or liberal eugenics[4]. In the current discourse, however, the concept eugenics in connection with the restriction 'liberal' is not only connoted negatively. Authors like John Harris[5] (2007), John Glad[6], Nicholas Agar[7] and Colin Gavaghan[8], to name just a few, promote liberal eugenics (often under the designation of Human Enhancement).

Among other things, Stratified Medicine is based on using genetic dif-ferences detecting parts of the population that, for example, respond specif-ically well or badly to a certain medicine or to identify populations that bear a special risk to certain diseases. At first this may sound harmless; however, old questions are raised again by those new opportunities of diagnosis: How to handle the information? How to avoid people being discriminated against because of that information? What are the social consequences of a "race-based medicine", for example?[9] What are the consequences of the early di-agnosis of genetic diseases for the unborn, their potential parents and those that are already suffering from the disease? What are the consequences of

---

[1]   The term "New Genetics" refers to genetics after the discovery of the double helix of the DNA.

[2]   M. Ekberg, "The Old Eugenics and the New Genetics Compared.", in: *Social History of Medicine,* 20/2007, p. 581-593.

[3]   T. Duster (Ed.), *Backdoor to Eugenics*, NY 2003.

[4]   J. Habermas (Ed.), *The Future of Human Nature*, Cambridge 2003.

[5]   J. Harris (Ed.), *Enhancing Evolution: The Ethical Case for Making Better People*, Princeton 2007.

[6]   J. Glad (Ed.), *Future Human Evolution: Eugenics in the Twenty-First Century*, Schuylkill Haven 2006.

[7]   N. Agar (Ed.), *Liberal Eugenics: In Defence of Human Enhancement*, Malden 2005.

[8]   C. Gavaghan (Ed.), *Defending the Genetic Supermarket: The Law and Ethics of Select-ing the Next Generation*, Abingdon/NY 2007.

[9]   D. E. Roberts, "Is Race-Based Medicine Good for Us?: African American Approaches to Race, Biomedicine, and Equality.", in: *The Journal of Law, Medicine & Ethics: A Journal of the American Society of Law, Medicine & Ethics,* 36/2008, p. 537-545.

the results of a genetic test for the individual? The genetic counseling tries to offer help in coping with the consequences last mentioned to those affected; however, similar to modern genetics, it has a partly dark history: the eugenic counseling.

2 Eugenics

The cliché of the eugenicist shows a misanthropic pseudo-scientist that is driven by racial hatred, being under the firm belief that the white "race" would be superior to all others and trying to breed a super race. Not only in Germany is the notion of eugenics inseparably linked to the Nazi policy of destroying so-called worthless life, with the nice and good-looking Joseph Mengele who is deciding between immediate and postponed death at the ramp of Auschwitz.[10] The eugenic policy enforced by the National Socialists determines the perception of eugenics in wide parts of the Western world. Eugenics is evil, bad, a combat term: whoever promotes new eugenics today can be sure of being closely linked to Hitler.

Nevertheless, there is not *one* eugenics but a great amount of differing eugenic concepts, which are articulated in varied historical, national and political contexts.

In order to answer the question whether eugenic ideals are still present today, e.g. in the context of genetic counseling, it is not sufficient to show that certain elements of the eugenic discourse can be found even today. Singular elements of a discourse do not have any significance of their own. For example, if someone positively refers to the notions of home and community, he cannot automatically be deemed a fascist. Fascism does not reveal itself by single elements. Those elements only become fascist by being articulated in a fascist way. The same applies to eugenics and the question whether and to what extent contemporary genetic counseling can be called eugenic or not. Eugenics has been articulated in different countries with different social, political and scientific circumstances. The political and economical circumstances influence the forming of theories and the reception within and without the original cultural sphere.

---

[10] E. Black (Ed.), *War against the Weak: Eugenics and America's Campaign to Create a Master Race*, NY 2003, p. 261-371.

The eugenic principles are neither bound to a certain evolutionary or hereditary model nor to a political system for their articulation. Nowadays, it is one of the common places of the history of science that there have been eugenic movements from the left as well as from the right. A less known fact is that eugenics does not depend on Darwinism but there are also Neo-Lamarckian articulations of eugenics and those that do not refer to genetics at all. To a certain degree Lamarckism is a better scientific foundation for eugenics than Darwinism.

Many works on eugenics start with the note that humans have been improving animals by selective breeding for centuries. As humans are mammals like dogs, cats, cows and pigs, they would be similarly modifiable. Whereas we pay attention to breeding plants and animals, e.g. records are kept and only the best specimen are allowed to reproduce etc., the human reproduction is completely uncontrolled, as the critics say. The American eugenicist Charles Davenport writes: "The eugenical standpoint is that of the agriculturalist who, while recognizing the value of culture, believes that permanent advance is to be made only by securing the best 'blood.' Man is an organism—an animal; and the laws of improvement of corn and of race horses hold true for him. Unless people accept this simple truth and let in influence marriage selection human progress will cease."[11]

The belief that humans can be bred is already found in ancient times ever since Plato. However, due to reasons of place and time, I will not elaborate on the ancient concepts of eugenics here. In the following, different articulations of eugenics will be outlined. The main focus of this account will be on Great Britain and the USA.

There is a differentiation between positive and negative eugenics: It is the goal of negative eugenics to reduce the reproduction rate of persons with "bad" characteristics and it is the goal of positive eugenics to increase the reproduction rate of persons with "good" characteristics. In general, negative eugenics is associated with compulsory measures like forced sterilization, prohibition of marriage or even killing. However, force is not a necessary element of negative eugenics. Many eugenicists rely on the reason of those affected, on their freely abstaining from reproduction. Principally, eugenicists, especially the US-American social reformers of the late

---

[11] C. B. Davenport (Ed.), *Heredity in Relation to Eugenics*, NY 1911, p. 1.

19th and early 20th centuries, would not oppose to enforce or recommend forced measures if those were beneficial to those affected or to the protection of society according to their opinion. "To understand them, it is necessary to recapture the mentality of a different world, a world in which even secular reform still retained a large dose of missionary fervor, a world that still believed in both the possibility and the desirability of benevolent paternalism."[12]

Positive eugenics mostly does without any forced measures; what is central here is the measure of appealing to reason and enlightening about consequences of dysgenic decisions. The greatest concern of the eugenicists of the early 20th century was the fertility rate that was at first glance very different in the different classes. According to the general opinion, the lower classes would reproduce much more quickly than the upper classes and the direct consequence of this would be that the upper classes would form a smaller and smaller part of the total population. Thus, above all, positive eugenics addresses society's so-called top performers.

Both forms of eugenics are necessarily judgmental; it has to be decided which persons are of good ancestry, which characteristics are favored and which methods should or, respectively, are allowed to be enforced for achieving the eugenic goals.

What is interesting is the fact that the history of science has mostly concentrated on negative eugenics. Even in 2001 Carson states[13] that there are no historical works on positive eugenics. In the course of the debate on the so-called human enhancement and transhumanism, however, it is increasingly referred to the historical predecessors of those modern movements. Authors like Julian Huxley, John Burdon Sanderson Haldane, both supporters of positive eugenics, and John Desmond Bernal represented those positions that nowadays are called human enhancement already in the 1930s.[14]

The eugenics movement in the USA can at least partly be ascribed to

---

[12] L. Zenderland (Ed.), *Measuring Minds: Henry Herbert Goddard and the Origins of American Intelligence Testing*, Cambridge 1998, p. 12.

[13] E. A. Carlson (Ed.), *The Unfit: A History of a Bad Idea*, NY 2001, p. 14.

[14] R. Heil, "Human Enhancement – Eine Motivsuche bei J.D. Bernal, J.B.S. Haldane und J. Huxley.", in: C. Coenen, S. Gammel, R. Heil, A. Woyke (Eds.), *Die Debatte über "Human Enhancement". Historische, philosophische und ethische Aspekte der technologischen Verbesserung des Menschen*, Bielefeld 2010, p. 41-62.

the so-called progressivism.[15] It was one of the main goals of this very heterogeneous reform movement in the USA at the end of the 19th and the beginning of the 20th century to improve the population's health.[16] It was not only the USA that was affected by heavy social issues and unrest at that time. The industrialization led to an enormous growth of the cities. The living and working conditions of many people were inhuman; tuberculosis, syphilis, alcoholism, malnutrition, contaminated drinking water etc. took their toll. In contrast to earlier attempts to improve the lives of the poor, the new reform movements referred to the knowledge and methods of natural and social science. It was typical of that time to claim to be able to solve urgent social problems based on scientific evidences (genetics, statistics, intelligence tests, etc.). Scientific solutions were very popular. In England and in Germany before Hitler's advent to power, eugenics can be understood as a reform movement whose goal it was not only to secure the genetic material but also to improve people's conditions of living. The eugenic movements were not only situated in a time of social unrest but also in a time defined by important changes in science: New methods were developed and old terms got new meanings.

The term eugenics was introduced by a British scientist, Francis Galton, in 1883:

"That is, with questions bearing on what is termed in Greek, *eugenes* namely, good in stock, hereditarily endowed with noble qualities. This, and the allied words, *eugeneia*, etc., are equally applicable to men, brutes, and plants. We greatly want a brief word to express the science of improving stock, which is by no means confined to questions of judicious mating, but which, especially in the case of man, takes cognisance of all influences that tend in however remote a degree to give to the more suitable races or strains of blood a better chance of prevailing speedily over the less suitable than they otherwise would have had. The word *eugenics* would sufficiently express the idea; it is at least a neater word and a more generalized one than *viriculture* which I once ventured to use."[17]

---

[15] A. S. Link, R. L. McCormick (Eds.), *Progressivism*, Arlington Heights 1983.

[16] M. S. Pernick, "Eugenics and Public Health in American History.", in: *American Journal of Public Health*, 87/1997, p. 1767-1772.

[17] F. Galton (Ed.), *Inquiries into Human Faculty and Its Development*, London 1883, p. 17.

In 1904 Galton defines the term as follows:

"EUGENICS is the science which deals with all influences that improve the inborn qualities of a race; also with those that develop them to the utmost advantage."[18]

The quotes show that Galton's definition of eugenics is rather wide; it refers to plants, animals and human beings. The goal of eugenics is to improve an existing population. This concept of eugenics does not depend on certain technologies and sciences, it only requires that a population can be affected pointedly, that plants, animals and human beings have characteristics that can be inherited by their offspring and that those characteristics' full development is affected by the environment.

But what exactly does "heredity" mean? At the beginning of the 20th century the term "inheritance" had a very broad meaning in medicine; it was not differentiated between "nature" and "nurture". A good example of this is Martin Barr, author of *Mental Defectives: Their History, Treatment, and Training* from 1904:

"Poverty, hard work, not infrequent intemperance, and many anxieties added to the physical sufferings of the period, might so press upon the mother as for the time to reduce her to a state of quasi-imbecility. If, added to this, she should have brought to her office of motherhood that exhausted vitality from a child-life in the factories, of which so much was heard in England, such a condition would provide fruitful soil for such a development of neuroses latent in the mother, as to constitute in her offspring almost a direct inheritance of defect."[19]

Galton introduced the differentiation of "nature/nurture" in its present meaning and he developed a new genetic concept under the term of "heredity" which differentiates between the influence of genetic material and environment. He writes:

"The interaction of nature and circumstance is very close, and it is impossible to separate them with precision. Nurture acts before birth, during every stage of embryonic and pre-embryonic existence, causing the potential faculties at the time of birth to be in some degree the effect of nurture. We need not, however, be hypercritical about distinctions; we know that the

---

[18] F. Galton (Ed.), *Essays in Eugenics*, London 1909, p. 35.

[19] M. W. Barr (Ed.), *Mental Defectives, Their History, Treatment, and Training*, Philadelphia 1904, p. 95.

bulk of the respective provinces of nature and nurture are totally different, although the frontier between them may be uncertain, and we are perfectly justified in attempting to appraise their relative importance."[20]

Galton ascribes a new meaning to the term "heredity", which was originally a term from the field of law and was introduced into the field of biology by Herbert Spence in 1863. Galton did no longer understand heredity as a vague, indefinite power as it was commonly done in the 19th century but as the physical transfer of core material which follows discernible rules.[21]

However, it would be wrong to state that eugenics has its sole origin in England. Even though Galton coined the term eugenics, eugenic movements were also emerging in France (*puériculture*) and in Germany (*Rassenhygiene*) at the same time.[22]

Galton preferred positive eugenics. "The possibility of improving the race of a nation depends on the power of increasing the productivity of the best stock. This is far more important than that of repressing the productivity of the worst."[23]

Such an improvement is only possible if those affected are successfully persuaded. Galton values eugenics extremely highly; indeed it would be a moral obligation.

Eugenics "must be introduced into the national conscience, like a new religion. It has, indeed, strong claims to become an orthodox religious tenet of the future, for Eugenics co-operates with the workings of Nature by securing that mankind shall be represented by the fittest races. What Nature does blindly, slowly, and ruthlessly, man may do providently, quickly and kindly. As it lies within his power, so it becomes his duty to work in that direction; just as it is his duty to succor neighbours who suffer misfortune. The improvement of our stock seems to me one of the highest objects that we can reasonably attempt. We are ignorant of the ultimate destinies of mankind, but feel perfectly sure that it is as noble a work to raise its level in the sense already explained, as it would be disgraceful to abase it. I see

---

[20] F. Galton, *Inquiries into Human Faculty and Its Development*, p. 131.

[21] R. S. Cowan, "Francis Galton's Contribution to Genetics.", in: *Journal of the History of Biology,* 5/1972, p. 389-412.

[22] W. H. Schneider (Ed.), *Quality and Quantity: The Quest for Biological Regeneration in Twentieth-Century France*, Cambridge/NY 1990, p. 4.

[23] F. Galton, *Essays in Eugenics,*London 1909, p. 24.

no impossibility in Eugenics becoming a religious dogma among mankind, but its details must first be worked out sedulously in the study."[24]

We have to do it because we can do it! We know that it is possible to improve the quality of the population by means of eugenic measures, in fact in a more humane way than nature can manage to. Galton concludes from this insight that man is obliged to take control. Eugenics should even become a religious dogma. Galton's idea that it is our duty, our destiny to control our genetic material is later taken up, among others, by Julian Huxley, the oldest brother of Aldous Huxley. He writes:

"It is as if man had been suddenly appointed managing director of the biggest business of all, the business of evolution – appointed without being asked if he wanted it, and without proper warning and preparation. What is more, he can't refuse the job. Whether he wants to or not, whether he is conscious of what he is doing or not, he is in point of fact determining the future direction of evolution on this earth. That is his inescapable destiny, and the sooner he realizes it and starts believing in it, the better for all concerned." [25]

At another point he writes: "The facts of evolution, once clearly perceived, indicate the position we men should take up and the function we are called on to perform in the universe. 'Stand there,' they say, 'and do thus and thus.' If we neglect to do as they order, we not only do so at our peril but are guilty of a dereliction of our cosmic duty."[26]

If man does not interfere and take control, we are threatened with downfall. The cultural achievements of mankind affect the genetic material in an unconscious way. What unites eugenics is the shared concern for mankind's future or the respective national population. Eugenics are reactions to social changes perceived as a threat: the growing impoverishment and massification of the population and the social unrest related to that, immigration, as well as – alleged – demographic asymmetries.

"The broad array of persons who considered themselves eugenicists shared a belief that scientific control over the processes governing human heredity would provide benefits to society. What such advocates meant when they spoke of 'control,' or of 'benefits,' however, differed markedly

---

[24] F. Galton, *Essays in Eugenics,* London 1909, p. 42-43.

[25] J. Huxley (Ed.), *New Bottles for New Wine, Essays,* London 1957.

[26] J. Huxley (Ed.), *New Bottles for New Wine, Essays,* London 1957.

from decade to decade, from country to country, and often from individual to individual."[27]

According to many but not all[28] eugenicists, a great problem was the repression of nature and thus accompanied by that the suspension of natural selection. Thus man would succeed himself to death by allowing those who would have no or only very little chance in the wild to survive and propagate caused by social progress (medicine, hygiene...). Culture protects the weak and thus harms the whole community in the long run. Since controlling the population is no longer in the hands of nature, man himself has to interfere and take control in order to counteract the growing degeneration. In 1923 Holmes describes the consequences of the "social betterment" for the human genetic material and thus summarizes the fears of eugenics.

"Civilization, biologically considered, is a comparatively recent and somewhat anomalous racial experience, and it brings in its train a number of agencies which tend to oppose the operation of those selective forces which most biologists regard mainly responsible for the evolution of organic life. Our modern warfare in leading to the elimination of our best stocks; our fostering of the weak and defective; the decline of the birth rate among those classes of society which have risen into the successful ranks, – all tend to recruit the next generation from stocks of relatively inferior racial qualities. There is little doubt that the most potent of these forces is the relative sterility of those classes whose inheritance of desirable traits of mind and character we have every reason to believe is above the average. In the animal world individuals that attain supremacy over their fellows generally succeed in leaving the most numerous progeny. But under modern social conditions this natural relationship between net fecundity and the qualities that lead to supremacy has undergone a curious reversal. Those who succeed leave few offspring, while the failures, the mentally subnormal and the improvident, who are restrained by no considerations of prudence from perpetuating their kind and leaving them to the tender mercies of Providence or the poorhouse, continue to multiply with relatively unabated rapidity. Whatever may be the forces working towards the improvement of

---

[27] L. Zenderland, *Measuring Minds*: Henry Herbert Goddard and the Origins of American Intelligence Testing, Cambridge 1998, p. 7.

[28] ... M. Pernick, "Eugenics and Public Health in American History.", in *American Journal of Public Health*, 87/1997.

our hereditary endowments, it is evident that so long as preponderating fecundity belongs to those who drift instead of to those who attain mastery the race stands in very serious danger of deterioration."[29]

Similar to Galton, for Holmes the threatening degeneration of society is rather caused by the refusal of the better-off to reproduce than by the high reproduction rate of the lower classes.

When comparing the definition of the American eugenicist Davenport in his book *Heredity in Relation to Eugenics*[30], which was important for the eugenic movement in the USA, with Galton's definition, it becomes evident that the concept is narrowed in its meaning. He only quotes the first part of Galton's definition "EUGENICS is the science which deals with all influences that improve the inborn qualities of a race"; thus he does not mention that "also with those that develop them to the utmost advantage" and goes on:

"Happiness or unhappiness of the parents, the principal theme of many novels and the proceedings of divorce courts, has little eugenic significance; for eugenics has to do with traits that are in the blood, the protoplasm. The superstition of prenatal influence and the real effects of venereal disease, dire as they are, lie outside the pale of eugenics in its strictest sense."[31]

Davenport does not deny that venereal diseases for example have dysgenic consequences, so that he recommends introducing a sort of health passport among other things. However, "real" eugenics only deal with hereditary risks. Leaving out nature as a *cause*, it sets the direction for the emerging American eugenics in an important way. Davenport points out: "It is the province of the new science of eugenics to study the laws of inheritance of human traits and, as these laws are ascertained, to make them known."[32] Davenport assumes that the actual causes of many diseases are genetically conditioned; however, they only break out under certain conditions. If someone has a nervous breakdown under stress, for example, then stress is just the trigger according to Davenport, whereas the cause lies in a genetically conditioned weakness of the nervous system.[33] Not all people

---

[29]   S. J. Holmes (Ed.), *Studies in Evolution and Eugenics*, NY 1923, p. 79-80.
[30]   C. B. Davenport(Ed.), *Heredity in Relation to Eugenics*, NY 1911, p. 1.
[31]   C. B. Davenport(Ed.), *Heredity in Relation to Eugenics*, NY 1911, p. 1-2.
[32]   C. B. Davenport(Ed.), *Heredity in Relation to Eugenics*, NY 1911, p. 4-5.
[33]   See C. B. Davenport(Ed.), *Heredity in Relation to Eugenics*, NY 1911, p. 254.

in whose bodies the tuberculosis agent is detected become ill, according to Davenport, but only those that have a special genetic disposition. "Rather, each of these diseases is the specific reaction of the organism to the specific poison. In general, the causes of disease as given in the pathologies are not the real causes. They are due to inciting conditions acting on susceptible protoplasm."[34]

The whole eugenic debate on nature and nurture is asymmetrical like any other debate based on polar dichotomy, one pole is more prominent. If accepting the differentiation gene vs. environment, the gene is always the basis as the environment can only affect something already present.

Davenport states that a genetic disposition does not have to come into effect depending on the environment or does not have any dangerous effects. For example, he assumes – like other eugenicists – that there is a hereditary "wandering instinct"[35]. Thus he writes: "Even the fugue tendency of the child of three years [...] might not have expressed itself so acutely had he lived in the country with freedom to wander widely at will instead of being restrained within the confines of city houses and narrow streets."[36] Furthermore, education would be important, yet again it would depend on the child's genetic basis whether he/she is able to learn quickly or slowly. Education can make the child's genetic endowment flower but it never leads to developing abilities that surpass it.[37]

Davenport assumes that psychic illnesses are not hereditary but the predisposition for such diseases is. This is an assumption common in medicine in those days which Davenport does not articulate like Barr mentioned above referring to Lamarckian concepts but following Galton, Weismann and Mendel. Already Galton deemed "nature" more important than "environment" for hereditary processes. Weismann's "germ plasm" which is passed on independently from body cells and Mendel's studies on the heredity of characteristics as discrete units led to the fact that the environment was deemed less and less important.

Apart from narrowing the view on genetic causes, British and the US-American eugenics can be differentiated by their setting of focus: positive

---

[34] C. B. Davenport(Ed.), *Heredity in Relation to Eugenics*, NY 1911, p. 253.
[35] C. B. Davenport(Ed.), *Heredity in Relation to Eugenics*, NY 1911, p. 90.
[36] C. B. Davenport(Ed.), *Heredity in Relation to Eugenics*, NY 1911, p. 253.
[37] C. B. Davenport(Ed.), *Heredity in Relation to Eugenics*, NY 1911, p. 254-255.

eugenics plays a rather subordinate role in the USA whereas negative eugenics has even influenced legislation. British and US-American society differentiate in their social structure and this is immediately reflected in their reception of eugenics.[38]

One of the most important critics of eugenics is Hermann Joseph Muller, who gave a talk on "The Dominance of Economics over Eugenics" at the 3rd International Eugenics Congress in 1932. Muller understands eugenics – especially its American form – as failure. As long as there were no equal opportunities in society, eugenic measures would not make any sense. Women, minorities and the lower class are always socially disadvantaged. Muller writes: "There is no scientific basis for the conclusion that socially lower classes, or technically less advanced races, really have genetically inferior intellectual equipment, since the differences found between their averages are to be accounted for fully by the known effects of environment."[39] Muller was a Marxist and he was – like J.B.S. Haldane and Julian Huxley – positively impressed by the development in the USSR. In his book *Out of the Night: A Biologist's View of the Future*, first published in 1935, he supports positive eugenics. The basis of his eugenic considerations is artificial insemination. He assumes that "in the course of a paltry century or two [...] it would be possible for the majority of the population to become of the innate quality of such men as Lenin, Newton, Leonardo, Pasteur, Beethoven, Omar Khayyám, Pushkin, Sun Yat Sen, Marx [...] or even to possess their varied faculties combined." H. J. Muller (Ed.), *Out of the Night: A Biologist's View of the Future*, London 1936. Muller assumed that an egalitarian form of society like communism would be more appropriate rather than a capitalist society built on competition and exploitation like the USA when realizing positive eugenics in a just way. What also becomes obvious here is that the question "What is good for humankind's future?" evokes completely different answers according to the political views.

Eugenics does not only deal with the value of differing social classes but also with the question of race. Eugenics and racism were often very closely linked to each other. However, racism is no product of eugenics which does not have to be racist. The statement that there are different hu-

---

[38] E. A. Carlson, *The Unfit* ; A History of a Bad Idea, NY 2001, p. 9.
[39] H. J. Muller, "The Dominance of Economics over Eugenics.", in: *The Scientific Monthly*, 37/1933, p. 40-47.

man races was a broadly accepted basic assumption of anthropology in the 19th and 20th centuries. It was argued about how to differentiate the races and which races were superior. Not only within the field of eugenics was it intensely discussed if racial mixture should be allowed and if the end of the white race was impending. Furthermore, it was not only skin color that played a role but various white races were differentiated too. In the USA the immigration of people from East European countries was regarded in a more and more skeptical way. It was assumed that the quality of the immigrants as a whole was declining as it was no longer the European elite immigrating to the USA but social losers who would be inferior due to their intelligence and their genes. Similar observations are even propagated today, e.g. in Germany. Racism has used biology for its legitimization, but it is not dependent on it.

As already mentioned, eugenic deliberations are not dependent on certain countries, sciences or political systems, they grow in almost every climate. There have been eugenic movements with differing goals, e.g. in the USA, in Great Britain, Germany, France, Russia and South America. At first glance one could assume that combining Darwin's evolutionary theory and Mendel's hereditary theory would harmonize with eugenic fantasies of breeding in a much better way than Neo-Lamarckism that is apparently less deterministically oriented. Though Lamarckism assumes that acquired characteristics are hereditary, that the environment plays an important role and that the genetic material can be influenced by changing the environment, still it remains important for negative eugenics that characteristics are hereditary and thus the easiest way to improve the gene pool is by restrictions of reproduction. Lamarckism can even be used more effectively when defending the *status quo* rather than Darwinism. When assuming that crime, alcoholism and general asociality are not only hereditary but can be acquired and are hereditary, it is clear that the poor are doomed to poverty, alcoholism and asociality by inheritance and thus genetically inferior to the upper classes. It is more difficult to give this evidence by applying Darwin's and Mendel's theories. Furthermore, eugenic measures, e.g. forced sterilizations, can be promoted by social reasons independent from any biological hereditary theories. Since the children of the poor do not have any future perspectives apart from suffering in misery, it is better for them to be not born at all.

The Neo-Lamarckism that dominated in France[40] and in wide parts of South America[41] allows environment to have a much more important role in the realm of positive eugenics. In the eugenic movement in Brazil, eugenics and hygiene were often equated: "to sanitize is to eugenize"[42]. Trounson characterizes the Brazilian eugenics in a literary report for *Eugenics Review* in 1931:

"Apparently the Brazilians interpret the word [eugenic] less strictly than we do, and make it cover a good deal of what we should call hygiene and elementary sexology; and no very clear distinction is drawn between congenital conditions due to pre-natal injury and diseases which are strictly genetic. Friction in the family, sex education, and pre-marital examinations and certificates seem to be the subjects of most interest to Brazilian eugenists[!], whereas genetics and natural and social selection are rather neglected; the outlook is more sociological than biological." [43]

Eugenics first of all means social and political policies and only secondly it means scientific theories.

It is also wrong to state that eugenic considerations are pseudo-scientific per se. This impression is mostly due to the successful efforts of the geneticists after the Second World War to separate the history of genetics from the history of eugenics. One example of this is the popular history of biology *Darwin & Co.: Eine Geschichte der Biologie in Portraits* by Ilse Jahn and Michael Schmitt.[44] The term eugenics only appears in the article on Francis Galton; the articles on the Nobel laureate Hermann Muller, R.A. Fisher, Julian S. Huxley and J.B.S. Haldane, to name just a few, say nothing about this topic though the authors mentioned are some of the most famous and most influential eugenicists of their time. Eugenics was a permanent feature in school books and scholarly textbooks, universi-

---

[40] W. H. Schneider, "The Eugenics Movement in France, 1890-1940", in M. B. Adams (Ed.), The Wellborn Science, Monographs on the history and Philosophy of Biology, Oxford/NY 1990.

[41] N. L. Stepan, "Eugenics in Brazil, 1917-1940", in: M. B. Adams (Ed.), *The Wellborne Science, Monographs on the History and Philosophy of Biology*, Oxford/NY 1990, p. 110-152.

[42] N. L. Stepan, "Eugenics in Brazil", p. 119.

[43] K. E. Trounson, "The Literature Reviewed by K. E. Trounson.", in: *Eugenics Review*, XXIII/1931, p. 236.

[44] I. Jahn, M. Schmitt (Ed.), *Darwin & Co*, München 2001.

ties' curricula and in a number of biological professional publications. Severe criticism against eugenics (especially against its unscientific excesses) was uttered by eugenicists themselves, e.g. by Huxley, Haldane and Muller, who were concerned about the reputation of eugenics. The danger that was threatening eugenics through "quarks" and overzealous supporters became clearly visible.[45] Among others, the Catholic Church and the famous anthropologist Franz Boas expressed their criticism against eugenics.

As has been shown, eugenics is a polymorphous movement that can neither be assigned to a specific political direction nor to a single policy and which must not be discarded as unscientific.

3 Genetic Counseling

Depending on the eugenic concepts referring to, the question whether genetic counseling is eugenic or not is answered very differently. The question whether genetic counseling upholds eugenic ideals or not, does not only depend on the interpretation applied for the concept of eugenics but also on what is understood by genetic counseling and in which context it is articulated. Resta distinguishes four models of genetic counseling that overlap content-wise and historically.[46] 1. Eugenic counseling: Its eugenic goal is to produce as many descendants as possible of the highest possible quality and to avoid offspring with hereditary defects. The counseling is directive, i.e. those affected are not only informed but also get recommendations on how to act. 2. The neo-eugenic counseling arises after the Second World War, it is non-directive. "In the practice of genetic counseling, it is our policy to inform a responsible member of any family with a counseling problem of all the facts at our disposal bearing on the issue. However, with rare exceptions, we do not attempt to pass a judgment as to the advisability of parenthood."[47] This model assumes that those affected will make the right decision and will abstain from reproduction if the risk is too high. 3. The medical model of genetic counseling concentrates on the

---

[45] See among others S. J.Holmes, *Studies in Evolution and Eugenics*, p. 194.

[46] R. G. Resta, "Eugenic Considerations in the Theory and Practice of Genetic Counseling.", in: *Science in Context*, 11/1998, p. 431-438, p. 431 f.

[47] J. V. Neel, W. J. Schull (Eds.), *Human Heredity*, Chicago 1954, p. 308.

direct consequences of a genetic predisposition. The result of such counseling, for example, could be to recommend a prophylactic mastectomy if there was a high risk of genetically conditioned breast cancer. According to Resta, the direct goal is to improve the health and well-being of the patient and not to improve the gene pool. However, such counseling can have eugenic effects too. 4. The psycho-social model: "Eugenics, and sometimes even medical, considerations become irrelevant or secondary, and the emphasis is on the complex psychological issues engendered by being at risk for or actually having a genetic disease in the family."[48] The latter model is predominant in the USA. In general it has to be doubted that non-directive counseling is possible at all since "the very existence of the service, which makes it possible to offer termination as an option in the case of findings of genetic disorder, somehow implies that those conditions are not desired by society."[49]

Even if genetic counseling functions in a directive way that does not mean that it aims at eugenic goals. Thus, genetic counseling does have eugenic consequences; however, it does not have eugenic ambitions as the question is not asked whether a decision implies positive or negative consequences for the gene pool. Its focus lies on the well-being of those affected (parents, future children) and not the general good of the nation or mankind.

However, genetic counseling takes place in very diverse cultural contexts. The practice of emphasizing the patient's autonomy and avoiding directives follows the tradition of the Enlightenment and presupposes a subject concept coined by a Western perspective which is not shared by all cultures; e.g. the direction of genetic counseling in China (at least till the end of the last millennium) is explicitly eugenic: "improving the population quality and reducing the population quantity"[50].

If describing all activities that indirectly influence the genetic material in a "positive" way as eugenic activities, the concept of eugenics is diluted till it can no longer be discerned since any normative relevance is taken

---

[48] R. G. Resta, "Eugenic Considerations in th Theory and Practice of Genetic Counseling."in: Science in Context, 11/1998, p. 433.

[49] R. Chadwick, "Can Genetic Counseling Avoid the Charge of Eugenics?", in: *Science in Context,* 11/1998, p. 474 f.

[50] M. Xin, D. C. Wertz, "China's Genetic Services Providers' Attitudes towards Several Ethical Issues: A Cross-Cultural Survey.", in: *Clinical Genetics,* 52/1997, p. 100-109.

away. Genetic counseling is not inherently eugenic but it can be used to enforce eugenic ambitions within a eugenic articulation.

Acknowledgements

I would like to thank Harald König, Bettina-Johanna Krings and Bernard Wunden for their precious critical suggestions and advice.

Patients' Self-determination in "Personalized Medicine": The Case of Whole Genome Sequencing and Tissue Banking in Oncology

Tanja KOHNEN, Jan SCHILDMANN, Jochen VOLLMANN

Abstract: "Personalized medicine" in oncology is currently gaining considerable attention and evokes a multitude of hopes. The identification of genetic markers enables more precise diagnosis, targeted treatment and more detailed information about prognosis. However, the new technological options in the context of "personalized medicine" are also associated with ethical challenges.

This paper deals with the ethical and practical challenges of informed consent in the context of "Personalized Medicine". In this article we explore the current practice of obtaining consent in the context of clinical research, which includes genetic analysis and the storage of samples for future genetic analysis, which at the time of tissue sampling cannot be specified. We start our analysis with the characteristics of informed consent as they have been developed with regards to medical research. Thereafter we describe the ethical and practical implications of "Personalized Medicine" interventions for obtaining consent, and current concepts of consent which have been developed especially in the context of biobanks. In the final parts of this paper we will analyse the current practice of consent to "Personalized Medicine" interventions in oncology. Following an analysis of the ethical and practical challenges of such practice we will suggest "dynamic-dialogical-consent" as an ethically appropriate and feasible approach to consent in the context of "Personalized Medicine" in oncology.

1 Informed consent as an ethico-legal standard in medical research

The demand for informed consent as a requirement for medical research has a long tradition which goes back to the beginning of the 20th century. The first known state regulation for non-therapeutical medical research was formulated by the Prussian Minister for Religious, Educational and Medical Affairs in 1900 and may be described as the state's reaction to public crit-

97

icism after harmful medical research had been performed on many people without their consent.[1]

Almost half a century later the Nuremberg Code (1947) was formulated in the course of the Nuremberg Trial on medical experimentation during the Nazi regime. The codex, which, in contrast to the early German regulation, gained international recognition, comprises ten points for the ethically and legally acceptable handling of research with human subjects. This document establishes the standard of informed consent given by study participants based on the principle of autonomy: information, competence and voluntariness.[2]

A third important milestone relevant to informed consent and medical research is the Declaration of Helsinki (2008), which first was formulated by the World Medical Association in 1964. Differing from the Nuremberg Code, the Declaration of Helsinki distinguishes between "basic principles for all medical research" and "clinical research combined with professional care". With regard to all medical research, the Declaration defines inter alia that the researcher has the duty to protect the life, health, dignity, integrity, right to self-determination, privacy, and confidentiality of personal information of research subjects. Furthermore, the possible risks and burdens during a medical experiment must be communicated to the research subject as part of the informed consent procedure. The use of human material and data for research purpose is only permitted after obtaining informed consent.

In summary, informed consent constitutes an essential basis of the subject-researcher relationship in modern medical research. Hence, no research can be made without informing competent human subjects about the purpose potential benefits and risks of the planned intervention and obtaining his or her consent. Informed consent requires medical researchers to share decision-making power with the research subject.[3] In the following,

---

[1] See J. Vollmann, R. Winau, "Informed consent in human experimentation before the Nuremberg code", in: *British Medical Journal*, 313/1996, p.1445-1447.

[2] See J. Vollmann, "Informed consent. A historical and medical perspective", in: A. Okasha, J. Arboleda-Flórez, N. Sartorius (Eds.), *Ethics, Culture and Psychiatry. International Perspectives*, Washington DC 2000, p. 167-188.

[3] See J. Vollmann (Ed.), *Patientenselbstbestimmung und Selbstbestimmungsfähigkeit. Beiträge zur klinischen Ethik*, Stuttgart 2008.

we will analyse the implications of technologies in the context of "Personalized Medicine" in oncology for the ethics and practice of informed consent.

2 "Personalized medicine" in oncology: New technologies and their implications for informed consent

The result of the Human Genome Project (1990-2004) heralded a new era for medical research and clinical medicine since it paved the way for medical technology which can develop and implement methods for analysing complex genomic data sets as well as edit bio-information. Nowadays, the possibility of (whole) genome sequencing offers insights into the DNA structure and therefore patients' predispositions for diseases. Especially in oncology, "Personalized Medicine" has fuelled high expectations as a possible approach to diagnosis and treatment which is based on genetic and further characteristics. Today, it is possible to treat patients with certain diseases according to the genetic structure of their malignancies and to stratify patients into risk groups with regard to therapeutic efficacy of drugs and the progress of the disease. However, genome sequencing and other tools used in the context of "Personalized Medicine" do not only bring insight into the specific DNA structure of the cancer. The results can also provide more information about patients' prospective health constitution and other genetic dispositions. In addition, genome wide association studies steadily generate new genetic markers which may have relevance for patients' health. Against this background it is common practice not to destroy the tissue samples extracted for the purpose of a genetic based diagnosis of a tumour but to store it in biobanks for the purpose of future research. This practice has a number of ethical and practical implications relevant for the concept of informed consent. In the following, we focus on three aspects: 1. the reporting back of research results to research participants, 2. the use of material and genetic data for future research, and 3. the protection of privacy.

2.1 Reporting back results of genomic analysis

Reporting back results constitutes an ethical and practical challenge relevant to informed consent because as part of gaining informed consent researchers and participants in the research may need to negotiate whether and which information should be disclosed.[4]

During DNA sequencing of the tumour, results can be found which are not directly related to the current disease. Accordingly, researchers and physicians are sometimes confronted with incidental findings which can have a clinical significance for patients. This means that the results of "Personalized Medicine" technologies may exceed the frame of the original disease and go further than the initially declared purpose of an investigative procedure. Patients do not merely get information about their current disease but also get information which is not directly connected to their current clinical picture. While incidental findings can also arise from other investigations (e.g. imaging) the challenge with respect to genetic information is that it usually refers to a probability or predisposition for a certain disease which may or may not come up in the future. In this context, one ethical question arising is that whether there is an obligation on the side of the researcher to feed back these incidental findings to patients. It is important to bear in mind that disclosure of genetic information may be associated with beneficial but also harmful effects. Furthermore individuals' preferences with regards to disclosure of such information vary.

Moreover, there is a debate whether patients have a right to refuse such disclosure of health related information. The right not to know in the field of genetic testing may present an ethical as well as a practical problem because this may be associated with restrictions on the capacity to plan for the future and manage future symptoms. The situation becomes more complex if the genetic information may be relevant to third parties who share the genetic profile with the patient.

Last but not least, reporting back health-related genetic information poses challenges with respect to risk communication[5]. In light of the complexity of genetic information and its relevance for health it is crucial to

---

[4] A. L. Bredenoord, N. C. Onland-Moret, J. J. M. Van Delden, "Feedback of Individual Genetic Results to Research Participants: In favor of a Qualified Disclosure Policy", in: *Human Mutation*, 32(8)/2011, p. 861-867, p. 863.

[5] See A. Edwards, J. Gray, A. Clarke, J. Dundon, G. Elwyn, C. Gaff, K. Hood, R. Iredale, S. Sivell, C. Shaw, H. Thornton, "Interventions to Improve Risk Communication in Clinical Genetics: Systematic Review", in: *Patient Education and Counseling*, 71(1)/2008, p. 4-25.

provide correct and understandable information. However, this expertise may not be vested in those health-care professionals who gained informed consent for a diagnostic procedure.

2.2 Future use of tissue samples

The future use of tissue samples presents further ethical and practical implications relevant to informed consent. The scope of informed consent usually refers to procedures which are taking place in the near future. Hence, the participant in human research is informed about the procedure and its potential benefits and risks.

In contrast to the aforementioned scenario research in the context of "Personalized Medicine" often involves future use of tissue samples. Such a practice is ethically challenging because of the lack of information. At the point of time biological samples are collected, it is not possible to give patients detailed information about the future projects for which their samples might be used. It may be argued that patients cannot estimate the implications of their consent, because they do not have all the relevant information. This lies in the nature of the current focus on genome wide association studies which are core to "Personalized Medicine". Patients will receive relevant information at the time of consent with regards to the current diagnostic procedure, but physicians cannot give reliable information concerning the future use of tissue samples and research projects in the field of "Personalized Medicine". Therefore, the estimation of future scenarios presents a problem to the information aspect within the procedure of informed consent.

2.3 Privacy and "Personalized Medicine" technologies

Further practical and ethical challenges with respect to informed consent and future findings arise regarding the protection of privacy of research participants. Privacy protection is an ethical obligation of researchers and *"they have everything to gain from implementing robust protection, which in turn may create an atmosphere of confidence and encourage recruitment and retention"*[6].

However, this ethical obligation may collide with the aforementioned aspect of feeding back research results to participants. In addition, the emphasis of protection of privacy may run counter to the possible benefits gained by the use of sample and genetic data.

The encryption and coding of genetic data is crucial to secure the privacy of research participants. Different biobanks and clinical research projects choose different ways of handling the storage of the sensitive data collected: One possibility is the complete anonymization of the tissue samples and genetic data. The anonymization of data means that any link between genetic information and other personal information of the research participant will be destroyed. A second possibility is to pseudonymize the samples and data. In the pseudonymization the tissue samples and genetic data are linked to an identifier which may be linked to identifiable data of the donor. Thus, pseudonymization enables the assignment of a tissue sample to the donor. In contrast, the anonymization eliminates any possibility of assigning tissue samples to the donor.

One relevant ethical conflict arises with respect to patient privacy and a possible obligation to disclose findings. Following anonymization, recontacting the patient is impossible. The conflict between these two obligations gets heated if genetic testing results have a clinical relevance for patients as well as those who are genetically related. Another ethical question is related to the gain from genetic information. In many cases, it is necessary to associate the genetic findings with clinical findings to use the full potential of "Personalized Medicine" technologies. However, this will only be possible in the case of pseudonymization. Therefore, the chosen mode of coding the data affects not only the privacy and interest in information, but also the potential benefit to "Personalized Medicine" strategies.

---

[6]   A. McGuire, L. Beskow, "Informed Consent in Genomics and Genetic Research", in: *Genomics and Human Genetics*, 11/2010, p. 361-381, p. 367.

3 Models of consent to "Personalized Medicine" interventions

Various models of consent have been developed in the light of the afore-mentioned issues and further challenges associated with the technologies of "Personalized Medicine" (i.e. genome sequencing and tissue banking). In the following we will describe two such models of consent, namely the models of "broad" or "blanket consent" and "trusted consent".

3.1 "Broad" or "blanket consent"

According to the definition of "broad consent" by Sheehan, if

"an individual gives broad consent to the use of their sample or data in future research they are giving permission for someone else, [. . .]. to decide how to use the sample or data"[7].

The model of "broad consent" is a diverge form of informed consent and is based on the fact that in genetic research, future studies and projects might not be planned or even conceptualized when the tissue samples are extracted. With a "broad consent", donors can agree with future use of their data in different research studies which are not related to the current disease. One argument in favour of "broad consent" is the potential benefit of biobank research and the loss of such benefit in the case of strict policies on consent in this context. Furthermore, Hofmann argues that

"Biobank research has further incited the issue of alternative forms of consent because strict consent requirements can be difficult to fulfil in long-term research projects in a field where new technology, new perspective and new research questions emerge frequently. Often it is costly and sometimes it is impossible to obtain renewed consent – for example, when donors of material are anonymous or dead".[8]

With regards to the ethical acceptability of broad consent, Hansson et al. argue that "broad consent" should be recommended in the context of biobank research. This argument is based on the opinion that genetic research can

---

7   M. Sheehan, "Can Broad Consent be Informed Consent?", in: *Public Health Ethics,* 4/2011, p. 1-10, p. 1.

8   B. Hofmann: "Broadening consent – and diluting ethics?", in: *Journal of Medical Ethics*, 35/2009, p. 125-129, p. 35.

be seen as a social mission and people often have a general interest in medical research as well as in medical progress. Based on this, people should have the opportunity to participate in research studies. There should be no restriction to permit people to give a "broad consent" to future use of data and tissue samples because this would tangle and restrict their autonomy, so

"it is a genuine way of respecting people's autonomy[9][...]. Acceptance of broad consent [...] implies a greater concern for autonomy than if such consents are prohibited".[10]

In comparison with the model of "broad consent" the model "blanket consent" is characterized by the use of tissue samples without any restrictions regarding to future purpose, scope or duration.[11] Through "blanket consent" donors allow with a single authorisation any possible use of tissue samples. The German National Ethics Council encourages that donors should have the possibility to give "blanket consent", because

"donors should be able to allow for the interests of research by giving a blanket consent to use, but should not be permitted to hand over control of their samples and data to someone else completely and definitively."[12].

In summary, there is significant support in the current literature for the model of "broad" or "blanket consent" and the use of genetic samples for uncommitted purposes and future research. However, "broad consent" is deemed acceptable if it is connected with a safe handling of personal information and if the research projects have only small risks.[13] In addition, the right to withdraw consent or review it should be provided.[14] Contrary to the concept of informed consent, the model of "broad consent" is characterized by less information given. The complexity of information is reduced

---

[9]   B. Hofmann, "Broadening consent", p. 125.

[10] B. Hofmann, "Broadening consent", p. 127.

[11] See J. E. Lunshof, R. Chadwick, D. B. Vorhaus, G. M. Church, "From genetic privacy to open consent"; in: *Nature Reviews Genetics*, 9(5)/2008, p. 406-411, p. 408.

[12] Nationaler Ethikrat (Ed.), *Biobanks for research. Opinion*, Berlin 2004, p. 60.

[13] M. Hansson, "Ethics and biobanks", in: *British Journal of Cancer*, 100(1)/2009, p. 8-12.

[14] B. Hofmann, "Broadening consent", p. 125.

and donors only get minimal information with respect to the use of their tissue samples.

3.2 "Trusted consent"

Next to "broad" or "blanket consent", the model of "trusted consent" is suggested in the literature as a further innovative approach towards consent in the age of "Personalized Medicine". Its concept is based on the claim for a new alliance between research participants, researchers, and a third party authority. According to this concept the researcher should work without restrictions which may be imposed by gaining informed consent. However, this does not imply that anything is allowed. Instead, the concept of "trusted consent" encompasses approval for a research project by a third party authority. This authority, for example a research ethics committee, should be composed of members with substantiated and appropriated scientific, bioethical and legal expertise, together with a sizable fraction of donor representatives.[15]

Furthermore, "trusted consent" is characterized by different procedural steps which should provide the donors with choices regarding the use of their tissue and with safeguards guaranteed by the third party authority.[16] According to Boniolo et al., "trusted consent" may be divided into six different steps: In the first step, donors have to make a decision regarding the future use of samples. The second step contains the decision on the degree of identification of the samples. At this point, donors can choose between an identifiable, anonymized, and pseudonymized procedure. The third step refers to a choice regarding the retrieval of information, and in the fourth step, donors can regulate who can ask for information. In the fifth step, donors can give their prohibition, permission, or restricted permission on the economic transaction. The last step contains the choice regarding the recipient of the economic transaction.[17]

The models of "broad", "blanket" and "trusted consent" are discussed frequently in the context of biobank research and healthy donors. However,

---

[15]   A. McGuire et al., "Informed Consent", p. 364.

[16]   See G. Boniolo, P. P. Di Fiore, S. Pece, "Trusted consent and research biobanks: towards a 'new alliance' between researchers and donors", in: *Bioethics,* 26(2)/2010, p. 1-8, p. 5.

[17]   See G. Boniolo et al., "Trusted consent and research biobanks", p. 5.

as we will see, much of the research relevant to "Personalized Medicine" is conducted as part of clinical research. This in turns involves patients who, in the case of cancer research, are very sick. In the following sections of this article we will first reconstruct current practice of consent in the context of such clinical research. This will be followed by an analysis of ethical and practical challenges. Based on our analysis we will conclude with a sketch of "dynamic-dialogical consent" as an ethically appropriate and feasible approach to consent in the context of "Personalized Medicine" in oncology.

4 Information and consent in the context of "Personalized Medicine" in oncology

"Personalized medicine" in oncology often involves cancer patients who participate in clinical research. In the case of acute myeloid leukaemia for example, aspiration of bone marrow and blood is performed to receive cancer cells. The procedure is necessary for the diagnosis and genetic stratification which in turns determines treatment options. Depending on the genetic make-up, patients may be recommended to undergo bone marrow transplantation.

However, besides for the use of samples for diagnostic purposes, patients usually also give consent to the storage and use of their blood for future research. This may or may not have to do with the present illness.

In the case of acute myeloid leukaemia patients are often in an emergency situation regarding their disease situation and mental state. The urgency of the disease requires quick diagnostic and treatment. In this situation, gaining informed consent not only for the diagnostically relevant genetic stratification but also for further storage and genetic research seems ethical questionable. This is mainly for two reasons. First of all, it is questionable whether a patient in such a situation is competent to make these decisions. It is well known that following the disclosure of a serious illness, patients are not able to take in and weigh complex information. Against such a background, doubt seems warranted as to whether patients with acute myeloid leukaemia possess the capacity to give consent for the respective research. The second challenge refers to information. As we have pointed out already, it is due to the nature of future research that little or no information on the use of the tissue may be given to the patient and thus it is often not even clear whether the future research will be relevant to the patient's disease. Against this background, one may question whether informed consent is at all possible in such circumstances.

In the light of the situation of patients in the context of clinical cancer research described, the models of "broad" or "blanket consent" seem little appropriate. In fact, patients, who lack the capacity to understand the information given, hand over great discretion to researchers with regards to the use of their tissue. While such proceeding seems research-friendly with respect to future use of tissue samples and storage in biobanks it seems that the rights of patients participating in the research and the interests of researcher, the pharmaceutical industry, future patients and other parties who may profit and benefit from such research are out of balance. An appropriate approach to consent in the context of clinical research and "Personalized Medicine" is one key to ensure a fair balance of the different interests.

The model of "trusted consent" may offer some improvement with regards to the aforementioned challenges; by involving research participants in the six different steps described above, they seem to participate more in decisions relevant to future research. In addition, the donor has the opportunity to withdraw from the research with genetic material at any time. Donors may also specify which research projects they want their genetic material to be used for and which information, respectively findings, should be reported back. This is based on communication between researchers, donors, and third party authority and creates transparency between all involved. However, as stated above, the model of trusted consent is restricted to medical research and is not applied in clinical practice. Nevertheless, this concept with its focus on transparency of the complexity of information presents a first approach for an application in clinical practice in the field of oncology. Based on this concept and the fact that the informed consent cannot measure up to the new challenges in "Personalized Medicine", we suggest an alternative concept for consent in the field of oncology, especially where "Personalized Medicine" is used, which we call dynamic-dialogical consent.

5 Dynamic-dialogical consent: A first outline for an ethical approach to "Personalized Medicine" in oncology?

As pointed out before, "Personalized Medicine" in oncology implies that many patients provide tissue samples which are not only relevant for diagnostics and treatment but which are also used for research such as genome sequencing and tissue storage. Therefore, there is a close connection between medical practice and research and patients participate in clinical studies while receiving treatment at the same time. This special situation and the complexity of information must be considered with regards to consent in clinical research and "Personalized Medicine".

As a minimal requirement for research which is embedded into the diagnosis and treatment of a life threatening disease, we would argue that any information about research and the gain of consent must be separated from information and consent for diagnosis and treatment related to the present disease. This demand is based mainly on the well known limitation to take in and weigh information in situations of diagnosis of life threatening illnesses and associated reduction of competence. In other words, any research related information and consent should not be combined with informed consent regarding the frequently urgent steps necessary to diagnose and treat the patient. In addition to the separation of research related informed consent we argue that there are approaches to consent for research matters which in our view are ethically more acceptable than "broad" or "blanket consent" in the context of clinical research and "personalized medicine" in oncology. We suggest a model of "dynamic-dialogical consent" which consists of two parts and which will briefly outlined in the following.

The *dynamic part* of this concept takes into account the new development in research which may make it necessary to use the obtained tissue in the future. According to this concept, patients who participate in clinical research initially give their consent to the specific diagnostic procedures relevant to their treatment. However, patients do not automatically give consent for the use in current or future research. If researchers want to use the material they have to contact the patient again and ask for permission. Besides changes in research the dynamic side of the consent model also reflects that patients at different times may be more or less capable to make decisions regarding the use of their tissue in research. In addition, it takes into account that at different times researchers are more or less able to provide detailed information about the planned research. The consent model is based on an understanding of patients as partners in the research process. Patients are given the opportunity to think about their consent for future use of genetic data and whether they want to know incidental findings or if they want to withdraw. It should be noted that the concept of dynamic consent is only possible on the basis of pseudonymization of data, because otherwise it is not possible to recontact patients. While this may mean that additional resources are needed for protection of privacy and to contact patients again, the approach may be also of advantage for the researcher. This is because this process enables the researcher at later stages to obtain additional health data from the patient which may be relevant to interpret genetic information.

The *dialogical part* of the consent concept is closely interwoven with the dynamical part. This is because both the dynamics regarding research development and the patient's ability to understand information implies a dialogue between researcher and patient. The dialogue part also refers to the idea that it is only the relevant or necessary information which is communicated at certain stages. The complexity of information regarding future use of tissue samples and possible incidental findings will be divided into pieces that are only relevant for a certain research situation. Within the dialogical process, the patient has the opportunity to ask specific questions about the research project and the physician or researcher can inform about the nature of the specific project, the purpose and the risks which have to be taken into account.

Clearly, the consent model suggested needs to be elaborated on with regards to a number of challenges. Such a challenge might be the question of possible delegation of consent to future research to another party. This is especially valid for "Personalized Medicine" in oncology because a proportion of patients taking part in clinical research will die before the time frame for research in "Personalized Medicine" has ended. Another aspect relevant to informed consent in such a context is that of the minimal amount of information which is deemed necessary to judge consent of patients as ethically acceptable. Last but not least the implementation of dialogical-dynamic consent depends on information technology as well as communication skills. From an ethical perspective such a process of gaining consent is not acceptable if the demand for dialogue between researcher and research participants would mean that too much of human and financial resources would be taken up to fulfil this task. However, given the technological development in other fields relevant to "personalized medicine", it seems possible that by means of technological support (i.e. decision aids) such dialogue can be supported and facilitated. Hence, even in light of the aforementioned and other limitations we would argue that dynamic-dialogical consent provides an ethically more appropriate alternative than "blanket", "broad" and "trusted consent" in the context of "Personalized Medicine" in oncology. The concept includes patients and research participants as partners who have the right to make informed decisions about their contribution to the development of "Personalized Medicine" in oncology.

"Everything Better than 50% Is Better than Now"

An Ethical-empirical Study of Physicians' and Researchers' Understanding of Individualized Medicine

Arndt HESSLING

Abstract: "Individualized Medicine", a paradigm of clinical research, has moved into the focus of attention. A socio-empirical interview study was conducted with members of a prominent German clinical research group dealing with implementing "Individualized Medicine" into the area of colorectal cancer. The interviews (N=19) were based on a pre-structured questionnaire. The goal was to get insights into moral and social issues related to physician-patientinteraction and clinical care from a physicians' and researchers' point of view. The analysis revealed a broad spectrum of opinions. Findings discussed in this article are categorized under a) dealing with false test results; b) changing the physician-patient relationship and c) sensitive data. According to our analysis, major problems will be uncertainties related to the sensitivity and specificity of biomarkers, the identification of 'non-responders', the possible impact on the physician-patientrelationship, the handling of sensitive data and the difficulty to enable patients to understand genetic test complexity with the aim of obtaining an "informed consent".

1 Introduction

Within the last years, the idea of "Individualized Medicine" has moved into the focus of attention. In particular, this is made plain by the number of publications featuring the terms "Individualized Medicine"[1] or "Personal-

---

[1] The phrases "Individualized Medicine" and "Personalized Medicine" are often used synonymously in a wide variety of medical research. However, both phrases are mostly used in the context of genetic research. Until there is no connection of the DNA of a human being and the situation of being a *person,* the phrase "Personalized Medicine" is seen as unfavorable. Therefore, we use the term "Individualized Medicine" to describe research projects with the aim of a genome and molecular based tailored medicine. See: R. Kipke (Ed.), *Mensch und Person. Der Begriff der Person in der Bioethik und die Frage nach dem Lebenrecht aller Menschen,* Berlin 2001.

ized medicine"[2] increasing exponentially since the end of the 20th century. At least 2012 of the 2634 pertaining publications contained in the U.S. National Library of Medicine were published within the last three years, 921 of them within the last year alone (23.07.2011). Both terms are being used within the context of genetic research (391 of the 921 publications) concerning pharmacogenetic testing and gene expression.

Pharmacogenetic tests and the analysis of gene expression are two examples of Individualized Medicine by means of genetic testing. While pharmacogenetic tests are used to predict a patient's[3] reaction to a specific medication[4], gene expression analysis can be used for prognosis[5]. Both kinds of information serve to specify the therapy towards more precision, creating less toxicity and adverse effects. At the same time, this specification is often applied to differentiate patients. In the case of Mammaprint[TM] by Agendia[TM], a gene expression analysis serves to separate patients suffering from breast cancer into two groups of high or low risk for future metastasis. According to this classification, a postoperative (adjuvant) chemotherapy is recommended (high risk) or not (low risk)[6]. A closer look upon the terms of "Personalized Medicine" and "individualized medicine" shows their rare use in combination with medical tests which are *not* focused on

---

[2] W. Fierz, "Challenge of Personalized Health Care: To What Extent is Medicine Already Individualized and what are the Future Trends?", in: *Medical Science Monitor*, 10(5)/2004, p. 111-123.

[3] In this paper the term "patient" will be used for both genders.

[4] U. A. Meyer, "Pharmacogenetics – five decades of therapeutic lessons from genetic diversity." *Nature Reviews Genetics*, 5(9)/2004, p. 669-676.

[5] S. Michiels, S. Koscielny, C. Hill, "Interpretation of microarray data in cancer.", in: *British Journal of Cancer*, 96(8)/2007, p. 1155-1158; A. Oberthuer, B. Hero, F. Berthold, D. Juraeva, A. Faldum, Y. Kahlert, S. Asgharzadeh, R. Seeger, P. Scaruffi, G. P. Tonini, I. Janoueix-Lerosey, O. Delattre, G. Schleiermacher, J. Vandesompele, J. Vermeulen, F. Speleman, R. Noquera, M. Piqueras, J. Bénard, A. Valent, S. Avigad, I. Yaniv, A. Weber, H. Christiansen, R. G. Grundy, K. Schardt, M. Schwab, R. Eils, P. Warnat, L. Kaderali, T. Simon, B. Decoralis, J. Theissen, F. Westermann, B. Brors, M. Fischer, "Prognostic impact of gene expression-based classification for neuroblastoma.", in: *Journal of Clinical Oncology*, 28(21)/2010, p. 3506-3515; J. Subramanian, R. Simon, "Gene expression-based prognostic signatures in lung cancer: ready for clinical use?", in: *Journal of the National Cancer Institute*, 102(7)/2010a, p. 464-474.

[6] G. Kunz, "Use of a genomic Test (MammaPrint TM) in daily clinical practice to assist in risk stratification of young breast cancer patients.", in: *Gynecologic Oncology*, 283(2)/2010, p. 597-602.

such a patient classification, e.g. regarding responsiveness towards therapy or likelihood of getting a specific prognosis. Interestingly, both terms are used rather infrequently for clinical testing which is actually focused on the patient as an individual in a strict sense, e.g. in the case of "drug monitoring[7]". Therefore, the terms of "individualized" and "personalized medicine" might be confusing to a patient.

The motive of many different research groups to establish an "Individualized Medicine" is the hope to tailor medicine, i.e., to find the right therapy for the right patient[8]. It is an effort to surpass the one-size-fits-all approach and to identify new ways to reduce unnecessary adverse effects. Oncology is one of the medical subfields where a lot of effort is spent on implementing an "individualized medicine" into practice. Different therapies in this field may cause a variety of different side effects such as Mucositis, Vomiting, Alopecia, Diarrhea, Nausea, Fever and Asthenia[9]. Furthermore, severe side effects like, e.g., myelosuppression[10] and gastrointestinal toxicity may be caused by neoadjuvant therapy of the locally advanced colorectal cancer (see below)[11]. These effects are particularly depressing if the patient does not profit from the received therapy. This burdensome situation is due to the current difficulties to foresee whether a patient is going to benefit from a therapy or not, creating a conflict of choice between quality of life on the one hand and survival time on the other. The current uncertainty leads

---

[7] Drug monitoring is used to gain information about the concentration of a drug within the organism of a patient. It is used when the given drug has only a small therapeutic range that is when the drug has a high potential of being toxic when it is overdosed. For example drug monitoring can be used for the chemotherapeutic drug 5-Flourouracil, see: M. W. Saif, A. Choma, S. J. Salamone, E. Chu, "Pharmacokinetically guided dose adjustment of 5-fluorouracil: a rational approach to improving therapeutic outcomes", in: *Journal of the National Cancer Institute*, 101(22)/2009, p. 1543-1552.

[8] R. A. McKinnon, M. B. Ward, M. J. Sorich, "A critical analysis of barriers to the clinical implementation of pharmacogenomics.", in: *Journal of Therapeutics and Clinical Risk Management*, 3(5)/2007, p. 751-759.

[9] A. Young, C. Topham, J. Moore, J. Turner, J. Wardle, M. Downes, V. Evans, S. Kay, "A patient preference study comparing raltitrexed ('Tomudex') and bolus or infusional 5-fluorouracil regimens in advanced colorectal cancer: influence of side-effects and administration attributes.", in: *European Journal of Cancer Care*, 8(3)/1999, p. 154-161.

[10] Bone marrow suppression, leads to a stop of the normal production of red blood cells. Bone marrow suppression can end lethal.

[11] M. W. Saif et al., "Pharmacokinetically guided dose adjustment".

to a general recommendation in favor of therapy, driven by the fear that a therapy which might be helpful could be withheld.

1.1 General ethical concerns discussed regarding Individualized Medicine

In terms of medical ethics, the underlying rationale of the current thera-peutic practice can be described as utilitarian: All patients receive therapy and the negative side effects in the case of non-responsive patients are ac-cepted for the sake of the "entire group". From an ethical point of view, it can be argued that "Individualized Medicine" by genetic testing opposes this current utilitarian principle and aims to minimize the number of pa-tients who currently receive an ineffective or unnecessary therapy. At the same time, the classification of patients with respect to their responsive-ness to a therapy or their need for a specific therapy will always lead to a number of false classifications of responders and non-responders (General fallibility of tests, probabilistic status of test results, insufficient state of the art)[12]. This point raises new moral concerns for cases where a responder is falsely classified as non-responder and thus does not receive a poten-tially beneficial therapy. Furthermore, future common therapies in oncol-ogy like chemotherapy, radiotherapy and antibody-therapies will probably be increasingly administered according to a patient's genetic classification which may result in a disadvantage for patients who are being classified as non-responders while there is no alternative therapy for their group. This is particularly troubling in the context of pharmaceutical research. If the causes for non-responsiveness will be found to be very heterogeneous, fur-ther research in this context and the development of specific drugs for cur-rent non-responders by pharmaceutical companies could be impeded[13] due to lack of possible financial gain.

---

[12] See S. Michiels et al., "Interpretation of microarray data"; J. Subramanian, R. Si-mon, "What should physicians look for in evaluating prognostic gene-expression sig-natures?", in: *Nature Reviews Clinical Oncology,* 7(6)/2010b, p. 327-334.

[13] See R. Kollek, G. Feuerstein, M. Schmedders, J. Van Aken (Eds.), *Pharmakogenetik: Implikationen für Patienten und Gesundheitswesen. Anspruch und Wirklichkeit der 'in-dividualisierten Therapie'*, Schriftenreihe Recht, Ethik und Ökonomie der Biotechnolo-gie 11, Baden-Baden 2004.

Research with patient's genetic data and the use of genetic diagnostics and prognostics regarding their ethical implications have been discussed for quite some time. Many publications focused on the situation of disease controllability and the stigma that might occur with the classification as a non-responder. An explorative study by Barnoy concerning the testing for a hypothetical late-onset disease showed that only a few participants would be willing to take a test that does not give an accurate answer concerning the probability of occurrence. Even fewer participants would be willing to take such a test if there was bad disease controllability[14]. Hedgecoe's study, concerning the topic of clinical genetic testing, showed that the potential of discrimination and the possible problems of informed consent[15] and patient autonomy arising from genetic testing are strongly correlated to the matter of disease controllability[16]. In an empirical study with medical physicians he also emphasizes that in the case of pharmacogenetical tests evaluating inherited information the whole scenario becomes more relevant for patient's relatives[17]. This would be particularly problematic in case the disease controllability was difficult. Hildt stresses that the moral concerns which arise from an "Individualized Medicine" by genetic testing are strongly related to the way of prevention that these tests are used for[18]. Prevention can be categorized into three different classes, primary, secondary and tertiary prevention. The goal of primary prevention is to keep an individual or a population healthy. By information dissemination, behaviors that are potentially harmful shall be avoided and beneficial behaviors supported. Secondary prevention is a form of early diagnosis: With its methods, e.g. breast cancer screening, diseases are detected at an early stage that

---

[14] S. Barnoy, "Genetic testing for late-onset diseases: effect of disease controllability, test predictivity, and gender on the decision to take the test.", in: *Genetic Testing*, 11(2)/2007, p. 187-192.

[15] "Informed consent" is a medical ethical term describing that a patient who gives his consent towards a treatment or a research project confirms that he understands the aims of the procedures, is free of external influences and capable of making such decisions.

[16] See A. Hedgecoe, "Context, ethics and pharmacogenetics", in: *Studies in History and Philosophy of Biological and Biomedical Sciences*, 37(3)/2006, p. 566-582.

[17] See A. Hedgecoe, "Context, ethics and pharmacogenetics".

[18] E. Hildt (Ed.), *Autonomie in der biomedizinischen Ethik. Genetische Diagnostik und selbstbestimmte Lebensgestaltung*, Kultur der Medizin Geschichte – Theorie – Ethik 19, Frankfurt a. M. 2006.

promises better prognoses or therapies than late diagnoses. Tertiary pre-vention is used when a patient is already ill. It comprises methods that are employed to slow down the progress of disease and to reduce the complica-tions of the therapy. Much bioethical research of genetic testing has focused on the means of primary prevention, whereas most pharmacogenetic tests and gene expression analyses can be seen as forms of tertiary prevention (even though they bear the possibility of primary prevention). The ethical relevance of genetic testing for tertiary prevention has not been in the focus of ethical research so far, but seems to be the major field of an Individual-ized Medicine by genetic tests. These means have not been in the focus of empirical medical ethics due to the fact that only a few pharmacogenetic tests and even less gene expression analyses have been implemented in the clinical practice yet. Rogausch and colleagues showed in their observations that many patients appreciated the possibility of taking such a test. They also found out that, while some patients were afraid of being classified as non-responders, doctors feared that patients would be stigmatized[19].

1.2 Socio-medical relevance of Individualized Medicine

Even prior to the advancement of "Individualized Medicine" by genetic tests, a rapid change in the appraisal of health and illnesses has already be-gun. Viewing the current standards of primary and secondary prevention, it is evident that the aim to diagnose and prevent diseases at an early stage has moved into the focus of health care services[20]. Accordingly, patients are be-ing held more and more responsible for their own health[21] while they often overestimate their personal benefit from screening methods such as, e.g., prostate or breast cancer screening[22]. Advanced research of "Individualized

---

[19] See A. Rogausch, D. Prause, A. Schallenberg, J. Brockmöller, W. Himmel, "Pa-tients' and physicians' perspectives on pharmacogenetic testing.", in: *Future Medicine*, 7(1)/2006, p. 49-59.

[20] T. J. Gates, "Screening for cancer: evaluating the evidence.", in: *American Family Physi-cian*, 63(3)/2001, p. 513-522.

[21] M. Grill, "Alarm und Fehlalarm", in: *Der Spiegel,* 17/2009, p. 124-135; Nuffield Council on Bioethics (Ed.), *Medical profiling and online medicine: the ethics of 'personalised healthcare' in a consumer age*, London 2010.

[22] See K. Kupferschmidt, Art. "Falsche Gewissheit bei der Krebsfrüherkennung. Die meis-ten Europäer überschätzen den Nutzen von Krebsuntersuchungen. Nicht alle Befunde

Medicine" is particularly interesting in the combination with the increasing range of prevention methods as it provides new chances of primary prevention, itself. Commercial companies like 23andme[TM] already offer healthy persons the possibility to send in one's genetic material in order to gain information about one's predictable risk to develop diseases like Diabetes or Alzheimer's using similar or even the same technologies that are used within the research of "Individualized Medicine"[23]. Until now, there is no clear recommendation how physicians and researchers should deal with results which are not the aim of research itself, but might be of future interest for the patient[24]. The new German Gendiagnostikgesetz (genetic diagnostic law) which was supposed to clarify the handling of genetic data, finally excluded legal regulation of the patients' involvement in the research process[25]. Therefore, it does not cover the handling of predictive information resulting from the research process. The parallel use of technologies which can, e.g., predict the risk of specific diseases or the responsiveness to a therapy in a commercial setting as well as in the clinical and research context underlines how important the use of genetic data has become and will be in the future. At the same time, the present patient's limited understanding of screenings emphasizes the need for an open discussion about the value and the risks which predictive information can carry for the patient.

1.3 The physician-patient relationship

The discussion about value and risks of patients' information becomes even more relevant when focusing on the physician-patient relationship. During the last fifteen years, ethical empirical research has investigated the physician-patient-relationship in more detail. Various studies showed that

---

werden richtig gedeutet. Es folgen Angst und teilweise unnötige Operationen", in: ZEIT Online 12.08.2009; R. Meyer, "Krebsfrüherkennung. Häufig überschätzter Nutzen", in: Deutsches Ärzteblatt, 106/2009, p. 1640.

[23] M. Evers, "Peepshow ins Ich", in: *Der Spiegel,* 23/2008, p. 154-156; X. Li, R. J. Quigg, J. Zhou, W. Gu, P. Nagesh Rao, E. F. Reed, "Clinical utility of microarrays: current status, existing challenges and future outlook.", in: *Current Genomics*, 9(7)/2008, p. 466-474.

[24] Nuffield Council on Bioethics (Ed.), *Pharmacogenetics: ethical issues*, London 2003.

[25] *Gesetz über genetische Untersuchungen bei Menschen* (Gendiagnostikgesetz – GenDG), Bundesanzeiger Verlag 2009.

patients often felt insufficiently informed about their disease. Particularly in oncological treatment, such a situation leads to patients' dissatisfaction[26]. Furthermore, patients increasingly strive for participation in the decision-making-process, particularly those who suffer from severe diseases[27]. Consequentially, an increasing number of initiatives have started to strengthen the patient's position within the decision-making-process[28] and to implement a "shared decision-making"[29]. Vordermaier et al., who evaluated the value of decision aids[30] for patients with breast cancer, arrived at the result that "patients who used decision aids experienced less decisional conflict and showed better long-term body image outcomes which were mediated by reduced depressive coping."[31] Empirical studies also showed that physician-patient-communication significantly correlates with patient's satisfaction[32] and quality of life[33]. Thus, adequate communication between

---

[26] A. Bredart, C. Bouleuc, S. Dolbeault, "Doctor-patient communication and satisfaction with care in oncology.", in: *Current Opinion in Oncology*, 17(4)/2005, p. 351-354.

[27] S. M. Dowsett, J. L. Saul, P. N. Butow, S. M. Dunn, M. J. Boyer, r. Findlow, J. Dunsmore, "Communication styles in the cancer consultation: preferences for a patient-centred approach.", in: *Psychooncology*, 9(2)/2000, p. 147-156.

[28] A. Loh, D. Simon, C. Bieber, W. Eich, M. Härter M, "Patient and citizen participation in German health care – current state and future perspectives.", in: *Zeitschrift für Evidenz, Fortbildung und Qualität im Gesundheitswesen*, 101(4)/2007, p. 229-235.

[29] Shared decision making is a form a physician-patient interaction that is especially focused on sharing information and being equitable in the process of decision making concerning the patient's diagnosis and prognosis. It pays practical respect to the patient's autonomy. See: W . . . Godolphin, "Shared decision-making", in: *Healthcare Quarterly*, 12/2009, p. 186-190.

[30] Patient decision aids are meant for patient involvement in the process of decision making. They provide information about the options and outcomes helping to clarify personal values. See: N. B. Leighl, H. L. Shepherd, P. N. Butow, S. J. Clarke, M. McJannett, P. J. Beale, N. R. Wilcken, M. J. Moore, E. X. Chen, D. Goldstein, L. Horvath, J. Knoxx, M. Krzyzanowska, A. M. Oza, R. Feld, D. Hedley, W. Xu, M. H. Tattersall, "Supporting Treatment Decision Making in Advanced Cancer: A Randomized Trial of a Decision Aid for Patients With Advanced Colorectal Cancer Considering Chemotherapy", in: *Journal of Clinical Oncology*, 29(15)/2011, p. 2077-2084.

[31] A. Vodermaier, C. Caspari, L. Wang, J. Koehm, N. Ditsch, M. Untch, "How and for whom are decision aids effective? Long-term psychological outcome of a randomized controlled trial in women with newly diagnosed breast cancer.", in: *Health Psychology*, 30(1)/2011, p. 12-19.

[32] M. E. Suarez-Almazor, "Patient-physician communication.", in: *Current Opinion in Rheumatology*, 16(2)/2004, p. 91-95.

[33] S. E. Thorne, B. D. Bultz, W. F. Baile, "Is there a cost to poor communication in cancer

physicians and chronically ill cancer-patients has a positive influence on the patients' health[34] and the economical aspects of therapy[35].

All these research results emphasize the importance of good patient information and physician-patient communication. The moral concerns raised by the introduction of "Individualized Medicine" and the increasing expectations towards the patient to be an expert of his own health accentuates the problems of this new technology for the relationship between patient and physician. In this context, we considered it to be important to obtain and record the concerns of persons dealing directly with Individualized Medicine and compare their views on the possible opportunities and challenges for the physician-patient relationship. Their confirmation or rejection of theoretically identified ethical concerns by experts familiar with these problems may shed light on moral problems of the actual practice and help to identify suitable solutions. This is the main topic of this study: to investigate the motives and the moral concerns of a research group whose aim is to implement "Individualized Medicine" by genetic testing for tertiary prevention. The focus is on the physicians' and researchers' concerns about the possible impacts of Individualized Medicine on the physician-patient relationship. This is one of the first research projects regarding the ethical aspects of Individualized Medicine in an empirical design focused on researchers and physicians who are involved in the research of Individualized Medicine.

2 Empirical Research as part of ethical research/Focus and data collection

Since this study aimed at exploring physicians' and researchers' reflections and motives concerning "Individualized Medicine", qualitative methods were chosen. Study subject was the international renowned clinical

---

care?: a critical review of the literature.", in: *Psychooncology*, 14(10)/2005, p. 875-884; discussion p. 885-876.

[34] J. Harkness, "Patient involvement: a vital principle for patient-centred health care.", in: *World Hospital and Health Services*, 41(2)/2005, p. 12-16, p. 40-43.

[35] C. Lehmann, U. Koch, A. Mehnert, "Die Bedeutung der Arzt-Patient-Kommunikation für die psychische Belastung und die Inanspruchnahme von Unterstützungsangeboten bei Krebspatienten. Ein Literaturüberblick über den gegenwärtigen Forschungsstand.", in: *Psychotherapie, Psychosomatik, medizinische Psychologie*, 59(7)/2009, p. 3-27.

research group KFO 179 investigating a gene expression analysis for locally advanced colorectal cancer[36]. The group is located at the University
Medical Center Goettingen and consists of oncologists, radiologists, pharmacologists, biochemists, geneticists, statisticians and computer scientists.
Its aim is the "individualization" of therapy for locally advanced colorectal
cancer[37]. More than 65 researchers[38] were actively participating in the KFO
179 while this empirical study took place. Currently, the German guidelines
for the therapy of locally advanced colorectal cancer comprise the application of a neoadjuvant[39] radio- and chemotherapy followed by operation and
an adjuvant[40] therapy[41]. The KFO 179 group was able to show differences in
the expressions of certain genes of patients who do or do not respond to neoadjuvant radio- or chemotherapy. Based on this possibility of differentiation
between responders and non-responders the further aim is to avoid unnecessary side-effects and to create a more precise specification of therapy. The
members were asked to participate in an empirical-ethical study. During
the study period, the KFO 179 was divided into 8 subgroups[42]. In analogy

---

[36] The colorectal carcinoma is the second most common cancer in Germany and the second most common cause of cancer related death. The locally advanced colorectal cancer
belongs to the category of colorectal cancers. The standard therapy for the locally advanced colorectal cancer includes neoadjuvant therapy, surgery and adjuvant therapy.

[37] http://www.kfo179.de.

[38] All staff members actively involved in the research process were counted as researchers,
whether they are physicians or not. Subsequently, we will differentiate between physicians also being active as researchers and researchers who are not physicians.

[39] Preoperative radio- and chemotherapy with the aim to reduce the size of the tumor and
the number of tumor cells prior to the operation.

[40] Postoperative chemotherapy with the aim to eliminate all cancer cells that are left in the
organism.

[41] W. Schmiegel, C. Pox, A. Reinacher-Schick, G,. Adler, W. Fleig, U. R. Fölsch, P.
Frühmorgen, U. Graeven, W. Hohenberger, A. Holstege, T. Junginger, I. Kopp, T.
Kühlbacher, R. Porschen, P. Propping, J.-F. Riemann, C. Rödel, R. Sauer, T. Sauerbruch, W. Schmitt, H.-J. Schmoll, M. Zeitz, H.-K. Selbmann, "S3-Leitlinie 'Kolorektales Karzinom' Ergebnisse evidenzbasierter Konsensuskonferenzen am 6./7. Februar
2004 und am 8./9. Juni 2007 (für die Themenkomplexe IV, VI und VII) S3-Guideline
'Colorectal Cancer' 2004/2008.", in: *Zeitschrift für Gastroenterologie*, 46/2008, p. 1-73.

[42] SP1 Gene expression analyses and Gene-Polymorphisms, SP2 Functional validation of
differentially expressed genes, SP4 Immuno-Pet, SP5a Micrometastases, adjuvant therapy, SP5b Mismatch-Repair-Genes, SP6 Toxicity and Pharmacogenomics, SP 7 Growth
factor signaling pathways, SP 8 Biostatistics, IT-Infrastructure, Data Management.

to Mammaprint^{TM} of Agendia^{TM}, one of the few gene expression analyses already licensed by the US-Food and Drug Administration (FDA)[43], the gene expression analysis KFO 179 aims for, will be called "Rectumchip" in the following. Our aim was to interview at least one member of every KFO 179-subgroup. 22 members of the KFO were asked for an interview and all agreed to participate. Postgraduates who had not had passed their 2nd medical state examination were excluded. Because of illness and actual scheduling problems due to clinical activities, three scheduled interviews were cancelled. Of 19 members of the KFO 179 which were interviewed, 17 were male, two female. Their professional experience varied between a few months and up to 30 years. The interviews were held between June 2009 and January 2010. Five participants claimed to be exclusively dealing with research ((R1-R5) Researcher), the other 14 ((MD1-MD14) medical doctor) claimed that their clinical work was more important than their research work. One of the interviews was held with two KFO 179 members simultaneously. The interviews were conducted by the author, Arndt Hessling, (18 interviews) and Silke Schicktanz (4 interviews) and took between 30 and 90 minutes. We used an open, semi-structured questionnaire, covering three main topics:

– *Attitude towards "Individualized Medicine" by genetic tests* (Importance of test validity, positive predictive value, negative predictive value, dealing with uncertainty and ignorance etc.).
– *Evaluation of the current patient situation and assessment of meaning of a genetic testing like a future "Rectumchip" for patients* (expectations of the patient, situation of medical research, achieving informed consent, respecting patient's autonomy).
– *Significance of a future "Rectumchip" for the physician-patient relationship* (potential new problems of achieving informed consent, neglecting of patients due to tests, patient autonomy, patients' perception of the physician).

After a pretest, the questionnaire was re-adjusted with emphasis on patient's advantages and disadvantages. The participants agreed to the interviews being recorded, transcribed and pseudonymized. The principles of biomedical ethics developed by Beauchamp and Childress had been used to

---

[43] X. Li et al., "Clinical utility of microarrays".

identify possible moral decision conflicts in the context of "Individualized Medicine" by genetic tests[44]. In this way, they functioned as a hermeneutic tool to identify ethical issues within the empirical material. These previous findings were used to create the questionnaire and to define a coding list by which the interview material was coded. All interviews were conducted in German. All interview citations used within this publication were translated into English, cited interview passages are marked by exclamation marks. The recorded interviews were transcribed word by word and analyzed according to the qualitative content analysis methodology[45]. This social science research method facilitates a proper, systematic analysis of spoken material, by analyzing and coding the messages of the interviews on the basis of justified, predefined categories[46]. The material was structured by six categories which were deduced from the questions of the questionnaire and from the answers given. These categories were *recent frustrations, dealing with false test results, dealing with new forms of uncertainty, implications for informed consent procedure, changing physician-patient relationship* and *sensitive data*. In the course of analysis, the categories were reviewed and, in certain cases, reconsidered, improved and abstracted. Atlas.ti^{TM}, a computer software for qualitative analysis, was used for coding the interviews.

3 Empirical findings in an ethical perspective

The result of the data analysis can be bundled into six categories, indicating physicians' and researchers' motives to implement Individualized Medicine into the form of genetic tests. The expected possible advantages and disadvantages for the patient, patient autonomy, informed consent and the physician-patient relationship are looked upon from a physicians' and researchers' point of view. In the following, I will focus on the second,

---

[44] T. L. Beauchamp, J. F. Childress (Eds.), *Principles of Biomedical Ethics*, [6]Oxford 2009.

[45] P. Mayring (Ed.), *Qualitative Inhaltsanalyse. Grundlagen und Techniken*, Weinheim 2007.

[46] M. Lang-Welzenbach, C. Rödel, J. Vollmann, "Patientenverfügungen in der Radioonkologie. Eine qualitative Untersuchung zu Einstellungen von Patienten, Ärzten und Pflegepersonal.", in: *Ethik in der Medizin*, 20/2008, p. 225-241.

fifth and sixth category: dealing with false test results, changing physician-patient-relationship and sensitive data.

3.1 Dealing with false test results

The first category of interviewed experts focuses on the matter of false test results and their consequences for the physician-patient relationship. Following the current standard recommendation for locally advanced colorectal cancer in Germany, all patients receive a neoadjuvant radio- and chemotherapy, providing that the health status of the patient allows it. With that, some patients receive a therapy that would not have been necessary or does not help to cure their disease while they suffer from its adverse effects. The future classification by forms of Individualized Medicine, such as a possible "Rectumchip", aims at solving this problem but will never be completely accurate. It was discussed in the interviews what value the test accuracy would have to achieve in order to motivate researchers and medical doctors to accept such a test in medical practice. Most of the interviewees requested the test to be very accurate. Individually, the answers concerning this problem were very heterogeneous. One of the interviewees mentioned that she would have a bad feeling if only one out of thousand patients was tested falsely.

"The standard has to be extremely high. I try to treat every patient as ... if he were a family member and therefore I want the optimum. If there were one out of thousand classified wrong it would give me a bad feeling. I know 100% is not possible but in 99,99% it really has to be right on the classification that [the neoadjuvant therapy] does not work for this patient." (MD 9)

Other interviewees mentioned that everything being better than the current situation would mean a progress.

"65% does not sound too bad. It is better than 50%. If I do have 65% percent I do integrate this into a prospective study. Knowing that we treat patients wrongly, patients who receive preoperative therapy over half a year and dying three month after the operation because of metastasis, knowing that we took quality of life, that we rather should have sent them home and knowing that they did not enjoy their life and died, I think everything better than 50% is better than now." (MD 3)

These different views were linked with the subjective perception of the severity of the adverse effects. Members of the group of researchers and medical doctors who stressed the importance of a very accurate test estimated the observed adverse effects as less severe, whereas the group whose members were willing to accept a test without a very high accuracy viewed the severity of adverse side effects as more problematic. One member who pointed out different cases of severe side-effects also hinted at the fact that a test with less than one-hundred percent accuracy could be used in future trials to improve the patient's therapy step by step (see above). With respect to the parameters of positive and negative predictive value[47], most of the interviewees mentioned that they would not want to use a test that does not have a very high negative-predictive value. This implies that they fear the possibility that patients could be falsely classified as non-responders and therefore not receive therapy that might be helpful, as the following citation elucidates.

"You do not fear to oversupply but you fear to undersupply a patient. And this is problematic as in the individual situation you do not know whether it will help or not. Would it have been better to use a neoadjuvant therapy or would it have been worse? Individualization is good but it bears uncertainty. It is all based on statistical analysis." (MD 7)

Most interviewees considered it preferable to have rather a test with a low positive predicative value than one with a low negative predictive value. Interview opinions that the negative predictive value of a test has to be higher than its positive predictive value, confirm a general fear of withholding a therapy that might have helped the patient.

3.2 Changing Physician-Patient Relationship

The physicians and researchers showed a rather paternalistic image with respect to the current patient-physician-relationship in the oncological set-

---

[47] Positive predictive value (PPV) is the probability that a condition occurs (e.g. the patient does respond to the given neoadjuvant therapy) given the device output for that the patient will profit from the therapy. Negative predictive value (NPV) is the probability that a condition does not occur (i.e. the patient does not respond to the given neoadjuvant chemotherapy) given the device output for that the patient will not profit from the current standard therapy.

ting. A number of participants mentioned that patients do commonly neglect their illness and often want their physician to make the therapeutic decision. MD 1 for example explained:

"85% to 90% say: ['proceed as you think it is the best.'] And if I would explain to them that we put their DNA on a slide and the tests tell us which therapy to use the patients will say: ['do so']."

Concerning the physician-patient interaction within an oncological setting, one of the KFO 179 members (R2) said:

"I worked with patients who received chemotherapy. My experience is that most of them want the doctor to decide for them. The patients were overwhelmed because they did not have the specific medical knowledge. The common patient wants to place the responsibility on the doctor: ['the doctor shall do what is best for me']."

The opinions on how a future genetic test like the "Rectumchip" might influence or even change the relationship between patient and physician differ considerably. It was mentioned in a number of interviews that such a future test might lead to a situation where physicians do not pay enough attention to their patient.

"Yes, it can happen that the physician will make it too easy for himself. Maybe he has too much confidence in the test and hides himself behind the test result." (MD 4)

Some of the interviewed members of the KFO 179 held the view that the physician-patent-relationship would not be changed.

"I don't think that many things will change. We check laboratory parameters every day. I don't think that such a test will bring us closer to a laboratory medicine." (MD 1)

Few of the medical doctors thought that the future use of genetic testing for an Individualized Medicine might lead to less insight for the patient concerning why he gets a specific therapy, to higher expectations towards the physician for choosing the right therapy and therefore to potentially problematic situations between physician and patient.

"The patient will be more dependent on the physician. The physician will accumulate knowledge concerning the prognosis. The patient does not lose autonomy, but

125

his position will also not be strengthened... I think that expectations of the patient will be incriminating for me if he did not understand that the classification is not 100% accurate." (MD 11)

A third group mentioned that it might be that an Individualized Medicine has a positive influence on the physician-patient relationship.

"I believe it will change to the better because this therapy shows that we do care for the patient." (MD 3)

The quotations show the very heterogeneous concerns regarding the possible consequences of an "Individualized Medicine" for the physician-patient relationship. Negative consequences particularly in the context of patient-physician communication were suggested as possible outcomes but altogether the possible future consequences are looked upon as rather positive than negative.

3.3 Sensitive Data

Most interviewees agreed that future patients will not refuse a "Rectum-chip" because of the possible misuse of sensitive data, but different reasons. Few of the interviewees mentioned that patients might only take the test because of their illness and would probably not agree to the analysis of their genome if they were healthy.

"We have evidence that the point of time differs. A healthy patient says 'I will never let this happen to my data' When the patient has something, his opinion will change rapidly. I think I would take such a test in case it has to be done to receive the needed therapy. I would not take such a test in case I was healthy." (R 1)

Other researchers and physicians emphasized that most patients were pretty careless in the dealing with their personal data in many situations.

"I think patients are surprisingly uncritical.... Patients do not consider what happens to their data. Maybe it is a general trend in society that people do not have a feeling for what can be done with their data." (MD 11)

All interviewees agreed that the protection of sensitive data such as patient's genetic data was important. They suggested that the misuse of such data by employers and insurance companies would be a "horror-scenario". Clearly, their dissemination could and would have to be prevented. Furthermore, it was pointed out that the patient's data would be protected by the German "Gendiagnostikgesetz" of 2009. Some of the interviewees mentioned their feeling that patients would not care too much about the protection of their data and that, therefore, the physician's and researcher's job to fulfill the task of data protection would be particularly important. It was reported that the KFO 179 would abstain from investigating the expression of a gene that was found to be correlated with the prognosis of Alzheimer's-disease. MD 5 said:

"We do abstain from measuring variants which could have consequences ... like variants which can show a predisposition for Alzheimer's-disease. ... If we carried through a genome-wide analysis, which we do not, you would have this [data] automatically, then you have to be aware of it."

In this context it became abundantly clear that the use of genetic material can create information which could be important to the patient himself as well as to his relatives according to the prediction of other future illness within the family.

4 Discussion

Our study shows – as far as we know for the first time – the views of physicians and researchers about possible influences of Individualized Medicine on the physician-patient-relationship. The current standard therapy was described by the different KFO 179 members as a decision in a state of ignorance. The motivation for implementing an "Individualized Medicine" by genetic testing is to reduce this current dilemma by classifying patients into groups of responders and non-responders to a neoadjuvant radio-chemotherapy of the locally advanced colorectal cancer. This approach distances itself from a utilitarian principle which aims at maximizing the common good and pays more attention to patients who do not benefit from the current standard therapy. The approach to Individualized Medicine must therefore be seen as an opportunity to reduce unnecessary treatment. This includes that professionals accept the challenge to reduce or withhold treatment and implies the willingness to lower the interdisciplinary struggle for the patient for his own good.

4.1 The positive and the negative predictive value as input for interaction between physician and patient

From a bioethical point of view, the positive predictive value[48] (PPV) and the negative predictive[49] (NPV) value of a future genetic test for "Individualized Medicine" are playing an important role in future application of such a test. Most of the interviewed researchers mentioned that they only wanted to use a test with a very low probability of wrong classifications. Additionally, it was more important to most of the interviewed KFO 179 members to have a test with a high NPV than with a high PPV. The low PPV and the NPV of the Mammaprint^{TM} by Agendia^{TM} show that the FDA has licensed a test with a high chance to falsely classify positive patients[50]. For this reason, many patients who are treated according to the test results will still receive an unnecessary treatment. The very high negative predictive value provides the near-certainty that patients who will not get treatment according to the test result really do not need it[51]. For this reason, it can be an important tool for patients and physicians to trust on. If a future Rectumchip was accepted under the same conditions as those for Mammaprint^{TM}

---

[48] Negative predictive value (NPV) is the probability that a condition does not occur (i.e. metastatic disease does not occur within a given time frame) given the device output for that patient is low risk. In this context, negative means the patient is a non-responder.

[49] Positive predictive value (PPV) is the probability that a condition occurs (e.g. metastatic disease occurs within a given time frame) given the device output for that patient is high risk. In this context, positive means that the patient is a responder.

[50] TRANSBIG study: The TRANSBIG study was an independent European validation of the MammaPrint® 70-gene signature on 302 node negative patients who were less than 61 years of age and did not have adjuvant therapy. Results of the study are summarized below: PPV and NPV may vary with prevalence of gene signature high risk or low risk. In this study there were 191/302 = 63.2% high risk patients. Metastatic disease within 5 yrs: PPV = 0.22 (0.16-0.28) NPV = 0.95 (0.91-0.99); Metastatic disease within 10 years: PPV = 0.29 (0.22-0.35) NPV = 0.90 (0.85-0.96).

[51] B. S. Wittner, D. C. Sgroi, P. D. Ryan, T. J. Bruinsma, A. M. Glas, A. Male, S. Dahiya, K. Habin, R. Bernards, D. A. Haber, L. J. Van't Veer, S. Ramaswamy, "Analysis of the MammaPrint breast cancer assay in a predominantly postmenopausal cohort.", in: *Clinical Cancer Research*, 14(10)/2008, p. 2988-2993.

mentioned above, it would produce a high number of overtreated patients as a result. Marx-Stölting addresses the problem of wrongly classified patients as non-responders[52] from an ethical point of view. This idea is shared by most of our interviewees, and seems to have been taken into account when establishing Mammaprint™ as well. Still, there is room for discussion. The Mammaprint™ is presented with the argument of a high NPV which spares patients with low risk of metastasis an ineffective therapy. In this rationale the very low PPV of the Mammaprint™, which leads to an oversupply of therapy for 7-8 out of 10 patients[53], is neglected. The KFO 179 members argue that a high NPV is needed to prevent refusal of necessary treatment. Considering all different arguments for the same aim in toto, it becomes clear how confusing these facts can be for the patient and even for the physician.

4.2 The physician-patient communication

From the preceding paragraphs, the importance of passing this information on to the patient and the explicit need for reflection upon a patient's "informed consent" becomes obvious. This point seems to be even more important considering the statements that getting a patient's informed consent to being treated according to test results might become increasingly difficult in the future. Several KFO 179 members linked this point to the patients' poor ability to understand probabilities, emphasizing that there is a special need of "informed consent" dealing with the results of genetic tests – an aspect already pointed out by Hedgecoe[54]. He argued that "informed consent" for using pharmacogenetic tests was frequently not obtained. Our results emphasize not only the need for an "informed consent" with respect to the testing itself but also in the decision to be treated according to the test result. Interestingly, the view that patients would prefer

---

[52] L. Marx-Stölting (Ed.), *Pharmakogenetik und Pharmakogentests. Biologische, wissenschaftstheoretische und ethische Aspekte des Umgangs mit genetischer Variation,* Berlin 2007.

[53] B. S. Wittner et al., "Analysis of the MammaPrint breast cancer assay".

[54] A. Hedgecoe, "At the point at which you can do something about it, then it becomes more relevant': informed consent in the pharmacogenetic clinic.", in: *Social Science and Medicine,* 61(6)/2005, p. 1201-1210.

to have and the therapy decision made by their physicians shared by many of our experts stands in strong contrast to other current empirical studies on patients' perspectives. According to them, only a minority of patients prefers a paternalistic physician-patient relationship and really does not want to know much about the process of diagnosis and therapy[55]. Moreover, other empirical studies showed many patients to be interested in information on diagnosis and prognosis, particularly if they have a very serious disease[56] This proves that the physicians' individual perception concerning patients' wishes to participate in the decision-making-process differs from current socio-empirical studies. It is questionable whether this was due to the patients included in the research of the KFO 179 being unwilling to express the same wishes for shared-decision-making as in the other empirical studies or due to the physicians' misinterpretation of these wishes. The possible meaning of "Individualized Medicine" for the physician-patient relationship was described very heterogeneously by different members of the KFO 179. Some of the interviewed KFO 179 members thought a test like the Rectumchip would have no influence on the relationship between patient and physician at all, some mentioned possible positive influences, others possible negative influences. One concern of the ethical discussion was repeated by some KFO 179 members: Individualized Medicine by genetic testing could lead to an automation of the decision-making process.[57] The interviewees also mentioned the possibility of disappointed patients' expectations towards an Individualized Medicine may result in a loss of confidence in the physician. This revives a concern which was formulated by Rippe discussing pharmacogenetic tests[58]. However, the possible positive influences of individualized medicine on the physician-patient relationship were seen as more realistic. The "Rectumchip" focuses on quality of life issues and if this can be made clear to the patient, it increases the chance that the physician's actions are viewed more positively than in the

[55] D. Klemperer (Ed.), *Wie Ärzte und Patienten Entscheidungen treffen. Konzepte der Arzt-Patienten-Kommunikation*, Berlin 2003.
[56] H. Breivik, N. Cherny, B. Collett, F. de Conno, M. Filbet, A. J. Foubert, R. Cohen, L. Dow, "Cancer-related pain: a pan-European survey of prevalence, treatment, and patient attitudes.", in: *Annals of Oncology*, 20(8)/2009, p. 1420-1433.
[57] See L. Marx-Stölting, *Pharmakogenetik und Pharmakogentests*.
[58] K. P. Rippe A. Bachmann, K. Faisst, W. Oggier, C. Pauli-Magnus, N. Probst-Hensch, M. Völger (Eds.), *Pharmakogenetik und Pharmakogenomik*, Bern 2004.

current situation. In this context, the possible positive aspects concerning pharmacogenetic tests which Rippe points out on a theoretical level were also mentioned by some KFO 179 members[59].

4.3 The legal framework

The increasing importance of data protection becomes clear within the context of a progressing "Individualized Medicine". In 2009, the German Bundestag passed the "Gendiagnostikgesetz"[60]. The bill's aim is, on the one hand, to define sensitive genetic data and, on the other hand, to clarify under which conditions specific researchers may carry out genetic tests which provide better protection and patient's care. Few interviewees mentioned the Gendiagnostikgesetz would protect the data of patients classified by a future "Rectumchip". This assumption is not entirely correct. In the current situation, a possible future "Rectumchip" is not even close to being approved. Therefore, all sensitive data are obtained in a research context. The future evaluation of a possible "Rectumchip" in the clinic will still be a form of research, as well. This is important because the Gendiagnostikgesetz does not cover genetic testing in the context of research. The fact that the KFO research group actively abstains from measuring gene expression(s) as predictors for Alzheimer's emphasizes how the members of this research project try to reduce possible problems with sensitive data. At the same time, this neglects the fact that some patients are interested in their data and might want to talk about their predictive value concerning the possibility of developing specific other diseases. The patient's demand of adopting more responsibility for their own health makes the usage of pre-

---

[59]   K. P. Rippe, et al., *Pharmakogenetik und Pharmakagenomik.*

[60]   "The aim of the bill is to determine the prerequisites for genetic 'investigation' and in the context of genetic 'investigations' made genetic analysis as well as determine the use of genetic probes and data and to prevent the discrimination because of genetically 'properties' to preserve the national commitment for the respect and the protection of dignity and the right of informational self-determination", .()*Gesetz über genetische Untersuchungen bei Menschen* (Gendiagnostikgesetz – GenDG), Bundesanzeiger Verlag 2009.

dictive data even more important[61]. Offering possibly relevant predictive data to patients whose data are used in research information could be one way to guide the process of "Biomedicalization"[62] in a professional way. Currently, the Gendiagnostikgesetz does not provide any orientation about how to deal with patients demanding results from genetic tests that were not the main aim of the research. Therefore, guidelines how to act in such a situation seem to be necessary. The Nuffield Council of Bioethics which partly discussed this problem in the context of pharmacogenetic tests concluded that the results of these tests should not be forwarded to relatives if they were of interest to the patient. It was only argued that providing individual feedback would be possible[63]. Since predictive data affect the patient as well as the physician and the patient's relatives, a structured handling of these information seems to be necessary. The importance of such guidelines is also emphasized by the patient's right to know and the right not to know, which might be affected, if his/her relatives want to gain information the patient does not want to have forwarded.

5 Summary and Outlook

Our research aim was to investigate how physicians and medical researchers who play an important part in the process of implementing an "Individualized Medicine" by genetic testing into clinical practice, assess

---

[61] See M. D. Bister, "Jemand kommt zu Dir und sagt bitte': Eine empirische Studie zur Gewebespende im Krankenhauskontext", in: *Österreichische Zeitschrift für Soziologie*, 34/2009, p. 72-78.

[62] "Biomedicalization is our term for the increasingly complex, multi-sited, multidirectional processes of medicalization that today are being both extended and reconstituted through the emergent social forms and practices of a highly and increasingly technoscientific biomedicine. We signal with the 'bio' in biomedicalization the transformations of both the human and nonhuman made possible by such techno-scientific innovations as molecular biology, biotechnologies, genomization, transplant medicine, and new medical technologies. That is, medicalization is intensifying, but in new and complex, usually techno-scientifically enmeshed ways" (A. E. Clarke, L. Mamo, J. R. Fosket, J. R. Fishman, "Biomedicalization. Technoscientific Transformations of Health, Illness, and U.S. Biomedicine", in: A. E. Clarke, L. Mamo, J. R. Fosket, J. R. Fishman, J. K. Shim (Eds.), *Biomedicalization. Technoscience, Health, and Illness in the U.S.*, Duke 2010, p. 47-87).

[63] See Nuffield Council on Bioethics, *Pharmacogenetics*.

moral concerns of this technology and think about possible changes within the physician-patient relationship. Moral concerns were voiced very heterogeneously within the interviewed group. Nevertheless, the answers regarding the potential meaning for the physician-patient relationship seem to be very valuable. Considering current problems of physician-patient communication, it seems questionable whether the expected possible positive changes for the physician-patient relationship are really achievable. The present difficult situation of communication rather confirms some physicians' view that by "Individualized Medicine" the distribution of knowledge might become even less balanced than it is in the current situation. Claiming the support of quality of life as one of the goals of "Individualized Medicine" becomes dubious, if patients do not get the chance to understand how terms like "Individualized Medicine" are used within the context of research and that it means nothing more than a numerically better chance to receive the right treatment. It also becomes clear that most of what is called "Individualized Medicine" is applied within the realm of research right now. Especially the legally unprotected situation of patients who are being treated within the frame of research projects emphasizes the importance of open physician-patient communication. Further investigations will have to examine the patients' views of "Individualized Medicine" by genetic testing.

The attempt to introduce an "Individualized Medicine" by genetic and molecular testing occurs while serious changes in the understanding of health and diseases take place. Technologies used by the research groups which try to introduce Individualized Medicine into the practice are similar to those being used by commercial firms like 23andme^{TM}. Such firms offer a direct-to-consumer "Personalized Medicine" by genetic testing. Patients can send their genetic material to these firms and get a prediction about their health risk with respect to common diseases like Alzheimer's and diabetes. Simultaneously, patients are increasingly held responsible for their own health. More and more medical screenings are recommended to prevent the manifestation of diseases. In this situation, it just seems to be a matter of time until the genetic prediction of diseases becomes a common tool within the soaring process of screening. A future medicine that wants to be "Individualized" also has the responsibility to inform patients about the risks that arise from getting information and knowing about possible disease prediction. It can be argued that research in the clinical environment has the duty to offer the patient at least the opportunity to understand the possible predictive value for other diseases that were detected in his tissue. In this context, it does become clear that Individualized Medicine not only changes the process of diagnosis and prognosis but also the attitude towards disease prevention. These changes require patients who are able to understand the implications of gaining information about diseases that might influence their future life. They have to be enabled to understand what a genetic test with a positive predictive value of 22% (as in the case of the Mammaprint^{TM}) means to their choice of receiving an unnecessary therapy that diminishes their quality of life. Representative studies[64] show that most patients prefer an open conversation about the uncertainties of therapy and that it is important for many patients to participate in the decision-making process of the therapy, especially in cases with bad prognosis and life threatening diseases. These findings emphasize that the improvement of physician-patient communication does not keep pace with the improvement of therapies and treatments. The results of this research may help to understand the possible risks of "Individualized Medicine" for the physician-patient relationship. "Individualized medicine" will not be really individualized unless a patient understands its meaning and can evaluate the possible risks of rejecting or confirming a medical intervention tailored to fit him/her. Therefore, the advancement of shared-decision-making in the context of "Individualized Medicine" is more than just desirable.

Our research shows differences in the physicians' point of view which are of further relevance for future socio-empirical research. Naturally, the patients' point of view is of interest in this context, as well. Especially their own beliefs regarding their capability of dealing with predictive information and their wishes regarding communication with their physicians about "accidental" predicative information are of high relevance and a possible target for further study.

[64] S. M. Dowsett et al., "Communication styles"; R. G. Hagerty, P. N. Butow, P. M. Ellis, E. A. Lobb, S. C. Pendlebury, N. Leighl, C. MacLeod, M. H. N. Tattersall, "Communicating with realism and hope: incurable cancer patients' views on the disclosure of prognosis.", in: *Journal of Clinical Oncology*, 23(6)/2005, p. 1278-1288.

On the Value of Privacy in Individualized Medicine

Arndt BIALOBRZESKI

Abstract: If the approach of Individualized Medicine shall forge ahead, several steps are necessary on its pathway. One of these steps is the integration of biobanks into the larger medical research infrastructure but there remain open questions how to build them up successfully and sustainably. Since patients usually have a personal incentive to contribute a tissue and data sample to a disease-oriented biobank indispensable population biobanks instead need to make significant efforts to generate enough donations. It turns out that privacy expectations frame both the hesitance of potential donors and the policy of population biobanks how to handle the donated objects and their delivering human subjects. Therefore, predominantly existing privacy concepts will be sketched out in order to illustrate why people highly value their privacy that possibly could be infringed by biobanks. Different relational models of individual and common interests are pointing out what ethical framework should be chosen since it co-determines a biobank's success and viability. As a result, it becomes clear whether population biobanks should opt for a liberal or communitarian framework, or even for a third way.

1 Introduction

Individualized medicine seems to usher in a new era of medicine, but lacks certain powers of self-assertion yet. In the long chain of entities and steps that are necessary for a pathway of implementing individualized medicine into the healthcare system, biobanks need to be developed as a key infrastructure, and sustainably maintained.[1] However, for several reasons the existence and success of biobanks and biobanking networks like the BBMRI cannot be taken for granted.[2] Among other important milestones, sufficient ethical frameworks are necessary that are capable of dealing appropriately with societal privacy expectations. In comparison to patient biobanks that usually can rely on the intrinsic motivation of ill people to contribute to

---

[1] See European Commission Research & Innovation DG (Ed.), *Biobanking and Biomolecular Resources Research Infrastructure. Final Report*, 2011, p. 4.

[2] See P. Dabrock, J. Ried, J. Taupitz (Eds.), *Trust in Biobanking. Dealing with Ethical, Legal and Social Issues in an Emerging Field of Biotechnology*, Berlin/Heidelberg 2012.

the research with donations, a population biobank business plan that is dependent on voluntary donations without any direct benefit will only work if the given institution seems to be trustworthy enough for pro bono contributions. This is not a minor issue, since the Special Eurobarometer 2011 indicates that there is a certain hesitance among Europeans about sharing their private data, especially in terms of genetic data: 88% would favour a genuine legislative protection for it.[3] However, many European countries are lacking such a legal regulation. Germany for instance passed a law on human genetic diagnoses in the year 2009, but intentionally disregarded genetic analyses for research.[4] Since then, German parties made legislative efforts to close this gap, e.g. with the launch of a biobank secrecy[5] that has been proposed initially by the German Ethics Council[6], but has not succeeded yet. But if people regard safeguarding regulations like, for instance, the biobank secrecy as necessary and biobanks cannot provide such regulations; people will not be willing to provide donations in great numbers. The importance of trust is usually underestimated, and trustworthiness of biobanks is hard to build, and quick to lose. If biobanks are failing to meet expectations of the society from whom they need to recruit, the donation rate would most probably drop down so that biobanks would finally fail to meet the expectations of researchers for being a valuable research resource, as well. In other words, biobanks can solve technical problems, but the really important task is to take up the societal challenges that are still slowing down the integration of genome-based knowledge into the healthcare system.

At the beginning, this article will describe the role biobanks are playing in the context of Individualized Medicine. Then, privacy problems will be identified to be one of the grand challenges of biobanking management. It will be illuminated how privacy conceptions are dependent on philosophical premises, so that it should become important to ask from what point of view claims are being made: from a liberal, or rather from a communitar-

---

[3] See European Commission (Ed.), *Special Eurobarometer 359. Attitudes on Data Protection and Electronic Identity in the European Union*, 2011, p. 3.
[4] See Deutscher Ethikrat (Ed.), *Human biobanks for research. Opinion*, Berlin 2010, p. 8.
[5] See   http://www.bundestag.de/bundestag/ausschuesse17/a18/anhoerungen/Humanbiobanken/1703790.pdf.
[6] See Deutscher Ethikrat, *Human biobanks*.

ian point of view? This illumination plays a fundamental ethical role since there is a *"challenge to all bioethicists: how to shift the locus of bioethical dialogue to bring to the foreground implicit assumptions that frame central issues and determine whose voices are to be heard, and how to sharpen the vision of a global bioethics to include the perspectives of the marginalized as well as the privileged."*[7] It will turn out that the reason for different emphases on privacy are different perceptions of the relation between the individual and the common good and different answers to the question which one is of higher interest.

2 The significance of biobanks for the success of individualized medicine

Biobanks play a significant role for the successful integration of Individualized Medicine into the healthcare system. They are part of a long chain of important factors that contribute to its success. If only one key part will fail, the whole chain will not work. Therefore, the so-called Bellagio-group tried to identify those key factors for a successful integration of genetic-based research into public health and how this process could be accelerated. Beside other important aspects, they are highlighting the fundamental role of genome-based science and its special technology (which includes biobanks) for the betterment of the population's health.[8] Several years later, a group of leading public health genomics researchers set a state-of-the-art global agenda for the successful integration of genome-based research into clinical practice. Again, a flourishing biobanking structure has been named as a core issue for generating evidences for an appropriate selection of measures:

"An infrastructure for population-based research that can systematically collect and evaluate relevant data to assess the impact of genetic variants (together with behavior, diet, and environment) on population health is urgently required, in the form of both cohort studies and population biobanks in developed and LMIC [low-

---

7   A. Donchin, D. Diniz, "Guest editors' note", in: *Bioethics,* 15(3)/2001, p. iii–v, p. iv.
8   See *Genome-based Research and Population Health. Report of an expert workshop held at the Rockefeller Foundation Study and Conference Center*, Bellagio 2005.

and middle-income, A.B.] countries, in addition to intervention studies that show health impact and clinical utility."[9]

Analysing the purpose of biobanks for the breakthrough of individualized medicine in detail, Angela Brand et al. are stressing in their report on the introduction of Public Health Genetics in Germany that it is not sufficient just to have biobanks. Instead, it is important to provide well-functioning biobanks that do not belong to a commercial setting. Without the provision of such a public infrastructure, it seems to be too challenging to study systematically the validity of susceptibility that would be helpful for epidemiological studies and public health.[10] But what is the view of the private sector regarding biobanks?

The pharmaceutical industry acknowledges the importance of biobanks as well. For instance, in a global market study of PricewaterhouseCoopers (PWC) 2005 on personalised medicine, biobanks are identified as one of seven key challenges that need to be met for a market success. PWC predicts that personalised medicine will fundamentally transform the healthcare system like the upcoming of antibiotics or the invention of vaccines, but at the same time PWC is aware of the fact that this endeavour faces several bottlenecks. One of them is the demand for huge biobanks that deliver the scientific resources they need for developing drugs. To their regret, the USA do not have any central biobank yet, where pharmaceutical companies could get information whenever they needed to. As a result, there is a lack of research material.[11] At the same time, they assume that the technological development, headed by the pharmaceutical industry, will raise serious questions. Whereas science and the economy drive the wheel, there

---

[9]   W. Burke, H. Burton, A. E. Hall, M. Karmali, M. J. Khoury, B. Knoppers, E. M. Meslin, F. Stanley, C. F. Wright, R. L. Zimmern, Ickworth Group, "Extending the reach of public health genomics: what should be the agenda for public health in an era of genome-based and 'personalized' medicine?", in: *Genetics in Medicine*, 12(12)/2010, p. 785-791, p. 789.

[10] A. Brand, P. Dabrock, N. Paul, P. Schröder (Ed.), *Gesundheitssicherung im Zeitalter der Genomforschung. Diskussion, Aktivitäten und Institutionalisierung von Public Health Genetics in Deutschland. Gutachten im Auftrag der Friedrich-Ebert-Stiftung*, Berlin 2004, p. 5.

[11] See T. Lefteroff, C. Arnold, PricewaterhouseCoopers (Eds.), *Personalized Medicine. The Emerging Pharmacogenomics Revolution*, 2005, p. 33.

are "*ethical and privacy concerns around gathering, storing, and using ge-netic materials*" [12] that slow down the process.

In comparison to the optimistic economic report, a technology assessment study of 2006 from the Office of Technology Assessment at the German Bundestag perceives a more complex situation that includes more critical insights than in the PWC report. After their comprehensive analysis of existing reviews about the scientific significance of biobanks, they conclude that the necessity of a thorough evaluation of their value for the public will remain, since lots of public money is spent for their endeavour and their long-term outcome is not quite clear. However, they still acknowledge that the research on the human genome has its own legitimation, because it is the leading discipline of the biomedically orientated life sciences, and maybe also of the medical research in general.[13] Two years later, the future report of the Office of Technology Assessment at the German Parliament on Individualized Medicine within the healthcare system confirmed the insight that the research endeavour is relying on multi-, interdisciplinary and international collaboration which has the opportunity to use an integrated research infrastructure that contains biobanks, storing large datasets and huge amounts of specimen.[14] Without biobanks, this research would not be possible, for instance regarding the testing of the validity of biomarkers.[15] To sum up, genomic research highly relies on the existence of large scale biobanks.[16] The problem is that their existence cannot be taken for granted, especially in case they are publicly funded and therefore depending on the benevolence of the public opinion since "*the rapid pace of change has produced two powerful, but conflicting, social reactions. On the one hand, there is very strong public support for breakthroughs promising better medical diagnosis and treatments, and for assisting with law enforcement (in-*

---

[12]   T. Lefteroff et al., *Personalized Medicine*, p. 4.

[13]   See C. Revermann, A. Sauter (Eds.), *Biobanken als Ressource der Humanmedizin. Bedeutung, Nutzen, Rahmenbedingungen.* Studien des TAB 23, Berlin 2006, p. 122-124.

[14]   See B. Hüsing, J. Hartig, B. Bührlen, T. Reiß, S. Gaisser (Eds.), *Individualisierte Medizin und Gesundheitssystem*, TAB-Arbeitsbericht 126, Berlin 2008, p. 13, p. 89, p. 111, p. 296.

[15]   B. Hüsing et al., *Individualisierte Medizin und Gesundheitssystem*, p. 208.

[16]   See A. Cambon-Thomsen, P. Ducournau, P. A. Gourraud, D. Pontille, "Biobanks for genomics and genomics for biobanks.", in: *Comparative and Functional Genomics*, 4/2003, p. 628-634.

cluding identification of missing or deceased persons); on the other, there are anxieties about increased loss of privacy and the potential for genetic discrimination, as well as about the capacity to regulate genetic science in the public interest."[17]

3 The intertwining of privacy expectations and philosophical assumptions

Regarding the usability of genomic based research, the amount of study participants needs to reach a certain critical mass. As pointed out by the Eurobarometer 2010[18] and the Special Eurobarometer 2011[19], there is evidence that privacy expectations, sometimes framed as a "trust" issue[20], need to be acknowledged in the context of biotechnology and biobanks. Otherwise, the recruitment which is a sine qua non for a well-functioning biobanking workflow process will not be successful, and an integral part of the supply chain for Individualized Medicine and public health genomics would fail. But why is privacy so important for people, and why is it also possible to value it in different degrees? The reasons are background theories that lead to different conclusions. Those theories will be illustrated in the following.

Privacy expectations are dependent on implicit philosophical assumptions. Privacy usually belongs to a set of individual rights that are defended by liberal thinkers against the government and a morally demanding or socially oppressive society. Since there is no consensus about a clear notion of privacy, it is necessary to distinguish several concepts with distinct features. Three important concepts will be investigated: The philosopher Beate Rössler presents a useful definition that stresses the ability to control three spheres in the own life. Firstly, it is the control about fundamental decisions that affect the own way of life, called *decisional privacy*. Secondly,

---

[17] Australian Law Reform Commission (Ed.), *Essentially Yours: The Protection of Human Genetic Information in Australia*, 2003, p. 33.

[18] See G. Gaskell, S. Stares, A. Allansdottir, N. Allum, P. Castro, Y. Esmer, C. Fischler, J. Jackson, N. Kronberger, J. Hampel, N. Mejlgaard, A. Quintanilha, A. Rammer, G. Revuelta, P. Stoneman, H. Torgersen, W. Wagner, "Europeans and Biotechnology in 2010. Winds of change?"; http://ec.europa.eu/research/science-society/document_library/pdf_06/europeans-biotechnology-in-2010_en.pdf.

[19] See European Commission, *Special Eurobarometer*.

[20] See P. Dabrock et al., *Trust in Biobanking*.

it means the ability to control the access to personal data, called *informational privacy*. Thirdly, privacy means the ability to regulate the access to the own home or private territorial sphere, called *local privacy*.[21] In terms of biobanking, decisional privacy is at stake if a donor loses control over what can be done with his or her tissue, and informational privacy is at stake if he or she cannot control the data flow of the relevant personal data anymore. Principally, the line between access and non-access, usually described with the dichotomy of private and public, can be moved, and is subject to societal deliberation. However, within a liberal society this line is principally constitutive for liberty, since it is the guarantee of having a safe haven that protects individuals from governmental intrusions. Without any privacy, a society refrains from the idea of autonomy and finally abandons the idea of liberty.[22]

Besides the attempt of Rössler to provide a general definition of privacy, Helen Nissenbaum offers a concept that has the strength to highlight a genuinely technological aspect of biobanks: digital data and their flows of information. Nissenbaum defines privacy as contextual integrity. That means that the flow of information is bounded to a specific context, and if the context is changing, the rules for informational flow are changing as well. Nevertheless, if someone does not adapt the own flow of information to a specific context and applies one that is different than the socially accepted in that area, the right for privacy is violated. In the words of Nissenbaum, the governing norms of distribution are not obeyed so that the contextual integrity of information is not preserved.[23] In the context of biobanks, this concept means that when biobanks are not anymore distributing personal information with regard to the expectations of donors, they are infringing their privacy rights and needs. As a result, this code of conduct would collide with well-established rules of a liberal society and could hardly get the approval of its liberal citizens.

In contrast to Rössler and Nissenbaum, the jurist Daniel Solove presents a fundamentally different account of privacy which is not characterized by one stable concept, but embraces many aspects of "privacy" that do not

---

[21] See B. Rössler (Ed.), *The Value of Privacy*, Cambridge 2005, p. 79-168.

[22] See B. Rössler, *The Value of Privacy*, p. 10-20.

[23] See H. Nissenbaum, "Privacy as contextual integrity.", in: *Washington Law Review*, 79(1)/2004, p. 119-158.

have a common signifier or an essence in common. Solove rather proposes to talk about a family resemblance of many different meanings of privacy, expressed with one single umbrella-term. As a consequence, he develops a helpful taxonomy that is not deductive like many essentialist privacy concepts, but rather seeks to identify typical circumstances in a personal life that are usually described as privacy violations, because they interfere with intended individual actions.[24] This inductive approach, especially developed for the 21st century, where societies are heavily driven by information and communication technology, allows to identify very precisely very new and diverse forms of privacy threats due to the technology progress, especially in case of the technologically driven biobanks.

Regarding the old and new sorts of privacy threats, it might be asked why people value their own privacy expectations higher than competing interests of others, especially if there are rational arguments that seem to let trump collective over individual demands. The deeper question behind the individual value of privacy is how the individual good implicitly relates to the common good that represents interests and expectations of the greater society. Unfortunately, very often the concept and value of the common or public interest is not explicitly explained, and in addition to this there is even "*certainly no consensus on the scope and limits of the concept nor often is it even clear what type of phenomenon is at stake – is it an objective, a procedure, or even a myth?*"[25] Usually, liberal thinkers are promoting the individual rights against the claims of society, best expressed in legal texts as a negative liberty, whereas communitarian thinkers are proclaiming values like solidarity and reciprocity that would consequently further the common good. Liberals focus on the individual and communitarians on the collective, so that both views could be understood as being dichotomic, but is this really the case? Are individual and common good mutually exclusive, or are they rather just different things that occasionally coincide? Or can they even be principally identical? Those three possible ways of understanding shall be further investigated in order to ascertain if a consensus between liberals and communitarians regarding biobank policies is principally possible.

---

[24]   See D. J. Solove, *Understanding Privacy*, Harvard 2008.
[25]   K. Simm, "The Concepts of Common Good and Public Interest: From Plato to Biobanking", in: *Cambridge Quarterly of Healthcare Ethics*, 20(4)/2011, p. 554-562, p. 554.

Having a look into the past, there are many examples representing each case. Thomas Hobbes, for instance, was convinced that in a state of nature the effort of all people to pursue their own happiness would lead into war, so that it would be in the interest of each of them to transfer their power to a central regime in order to pacify the state of nature. As a result, everything the sovereign does in favour of the people is in the interest of each individual.[26] For Adam Smith, the common or public interest was served best if people followed their own interests. Due to his idea of the invisible hand of God, the pursuit of individual interests automatically resulted in strengthening the common good.[27] In comparison to this assumed identity of individual and common good, Plato and Aristotle were convinced that the identity of individual and common good are different things that occasionally or at least in the long-run coincide, because the common good always serves the individual good since it serves everybody with cohesion, equality and justice.[28] Very different to that, Francis Bacon understood the individual and common good as mutual exclusive. Both are independent forces that will never reconcile with each other, even if selfish interests turn out to be of common interest. Weighing against each other, the common good is favourable. Therefore, in his view, it is a duty or virtue to strive for the common good even though it is against the own individual interests.[29] Surprisingly, even though Francis Bacon is historically very unique with that opinion, his kind of view can be found very often in bioethical discourses, as it will be elucidated in the following analysis.[30]

Having a more current look on the issue of individual and common interests, Vilhjálmur Árnason analyses the bioethical discourse on biobanking philosophically and detects two major lines of argumentations in bioethics that are claiming a strong tension between both interests: First, a narrow individual consent protects private rights at the cost of common interests.

---

[26] See T. Hobbes, *Philosophical Rudiments Concerning Government and Society [De Cive]*. Edited by W. Molesworth [1841], London 1641.

[27] See A. Smith (Ed.), *An Inquiry into the Nature and Causes of the Wealth of Nations*, London/NY 1964.

[28] See R. Herzog, Art. "Gemeinwohl", in: J. Ritter (Ed.), *Historisches Wörterbuch der Philosophie*, Volume 3, Basel 1974, p. 248-258, p. 248 f.

[29] See R. Herzog, Art. "Gemeinwohl", p. 254.

[30] See V. Árnason, "Database Research: Public and Private Interests", in: *Cambridge Quarterly of Healthcare Ethics*, 20(4)/2011, p. 563-571.

Second, a broad or even unrestricted consent disregards individual interests. By contrast, Árnason proposes a model that rather identifies a unity of both as long as citizens have a certain scientific literacy. The common bioethical view regards people as passive objects who either follow their individual interests by demanding restrictive consent forms, or promote broad consents that serve communal interests while downplaying individual interests of protection. But in Árnasons view, the ideal citizen is an active one that knows about the necessities of medical research and therefore intends to contribute to it with his or her tissue donation and information delivery. At this point, individual and common good seem to be identical. However, investigating the arguments for participation, he is quite unsure if genomics research infrastructures like biobanks meet the common good criteria. Neither are non-health-related welfare benefits a unique selling point of genomic research because there are a lot of other ways for providing jobs for young scientists and commercial pathways for companies. Nor are the health-related welfare benefits clear since there are still alternative ways of improving the healthcare system and providing a common good. A new focus on genetic determinants and disease risks, for instance, could be problematic because it would put new pressure on individual responsibility instead of reminding people of the joint responsibility e.g. for providing better working conditions. Moreover, the outcome of genetic research is not worth the costs, because genetic diseases can be detected by heritage as well. This system of detection is already able to convince people to change their lifestyle in order to improve their own health.[31]

In comparison to Árnason who expects an occasional coincidence of individual and common interest but questions the assumption that biobanks are meeting the common good criteria, the philosopher Ruth Chadwick is convinced that biobanks per se are striving for the common good. Chadwick, who promotes communitarian thinking within the biobank ELSI discourse, belongs to the category where the individual and common interests occasionally coincide, since she argues for a new emphasis on collective values like reciprocity, mutuality, solidarity, citizenry and universality.[32] In case of doubt, she would favour the common interest, lowering down indi-

---

[31] See V. Árnason, "Database Research".
[32] See B. Knoppers, R. Chadwick, "Human Genetic Research. Emerging Trends in Ethics.", in: *Nature Reviews Genetics,* 6/2005, p. 75-79.

vidual rights and interests because "*there is a duty to participate in research that could move medicine forwards on the basis of solidarity. It is questionable whether individuals should be free, from an ethical point of view, to refuse to help in an effort to relieve suffering for what could be regarded as trivial reasons, such as refusing to allow samples to be reused for research on drug abuse because of the disapproval of drug users.*"[33] Chadwick notices that new technologies are appearing that make new medical research and in the long run probably better medical treatment possible. Those kind of societal and technological advancements contain new ways of looking on things and make new ethical judgements necessary. If, for example, privacy and confidentiality cannot be guaranteed anymore[34], old ethical principles should be abandoned since they do not seem to work anymore. So in her view, the so-called communitarian turn did not happen due to certain powerful interests, but because of the old individual-centred ethical principles that simply did not work anymore. Moreover, she tries to remind the reader that every ethical framework stresses certain values and that it is acceptable that new values are downplaying the emphasis of other probably important values. She therefore exercises a new communitarian ethical thinking that even "*draw[s] on pre-existing traditions of thought [... that] may have had less emphasis in bioethics to date.*"[35] Comparing the three different approaches of the relation between individual and common interests it turns out that the choice between these three models generates an ethical framework that affects the policy practice of biobanks, most obviously in the choice of consent form, singled out from a whole range of existing forms. So, if a practice of biobank is successful, the ethical framework is one of the main reasons for its success, since the policy is the expression of its ethical framework.

---

[33] R. Chadwick, K. Berg, "Solidarity and equity. New ethical frameworks for genetic databases", in: *Nature Reviews Genetics,* 2/2011, p. 318-321, p. 321.

[34] See J. E. Lunshof, R. Chadwick, G. M. Church, "Hippocrates revisited? Old ideals and new realities", in: *Genomic Medicine,* 2(1-2)/2008, p. 1-3.

[35] R. Chadwick, "The Communitarian Turn. Myth or Reality?", in: *Cambridge Quarterly of Healthcare Ethics,* 20(4)/2011, p. 546-553, p. 550.

4 The ethical framework as a key factor for a biobank's sustainable success

Raising the question what kind of ethical framework co-determines the success of a population based biobank, it makes sense to compare representative biobanks that contributed significantly to the worldwide genomic research due to its size, complexity and overall professional effort.

The Estonian Genome Project, later called Estonian Genome Centre, started with a liberal, individual-centred framework, but failed to reach its self-set goals. At the beginning they refrained from the option to use altruistic arguments, and offered instead an individual benefit in form of a feedback on the generated genetic data. It turned out that at the beginning, over 90% of the population conveyed interest in the participation incentive, the so-called personal gene card. But in the end, there have not been enough participants so that they changed their rhetoric to more communal arguments like benefits for public health, progress of medical research, awareness of Estonia itself, economic growth, and being useful to others. By that turn, they were more successful than under the conditions of the former ethical framework. Likewise, their funding changed: Starting originally as a public-private-partnership, they are now fully publicly funded.[36]

By contrast, the UK Biobank focused in its rhetoric on the public good from the very beginning. They tried to engage people by spinning-off a public discourse in order to communicate values similar to communitarian values, stressing future public health benefits, (genetic) citizenship, solidarity, altruism.[37] They presented themselves as a steward of the public good, and promised to put the results into the public sphere.[38] As a result, they reached their goal of half a million donors faster than expected, even one and a half years ahead.[39] However, even though it looks like communitarian

---

[36] K. Simm, "The Concepts of Common Good and Public Interest: From Plato to Biobanking", in: *Cambridge Quarterly of Healthcare Ethics*, 20(4)/2011, p. 554-562.

[37] See N. Kanellopoulou, "Reciprocity, trust, and public interest in research biobanking: in search of a balance.", in: C. Lenk, N. Hoppe, K. Beier, C. Wiesemann (Eds.), *Human Tissue Research: A European Perspective on the Ethical and Legal Challenges*, Oxford 2011; p. 45-53.

[38] K. Simm, "The Concepts of Common Good and Public Interest".

[39] See T. A. Manolio, R. Collins, "Enhancing the feasibility of large cohort studies.", in: *Journal of the American Medical Association*, 304(20)/2010, p. 2290-2291.

values that have been stressed in the UK Biobank framework seem to be the reason for success, there have also been elements that usually belong to a liberal agenda: respect for persons meaning that their dignity is uphold and that they are treated as ends in themselves and not as a mere instrument. The idea of respect has been supported by secondary principles like privacy, confidentiality and non-discrimination, finally culminating in the consent practice. Regarding this, policy donors had to be protected, their commitments honoured, and researchers were forced to comply with the will expressed in consent forms.[40] Thus, people have been confident in contributing to the community by delivering donations and sensitive data, based on an intertwined policy of communitarian and liberal values: motivating people to serve the larger group they are part of, and downsizing their concern about privacy by the institutional integration of safeguards like a clear code of conduct for researchers to respect people's will.

As a result of this empirical observation, it can be concluded that only a mixture of a liberal and communitarian framework can guarantee a high participation rate. It should not be thought of both ethical frameworks as a logic in terms of either/or, but as a logic of both/and. This more balanced approach fosters the strengths of both ethical frameworks with regard of donation motivation and need for privacy and control, and reduces the potential detriments of impairing the dignity and leaving potential medical progress unexploited. Irrespective of the question whether individualized medicine will develop the power of self-assertion in modern health care, at least population biobanks will contribute their deliverables for this endeavour, if they assume an obligation for the privacy concerns of donors and the trustworthiness of themselves so that individual and common interests not only occasionally, but intentionally coincide.

Acknowledgments

This work is part of the research program "PRIVATE Gen. Privacy Regimes Investigated: Variations, Adaptations, and Transformations in an Era of (post-) Genomics" (www.private-gen.eu), which is funded by the German

---

40 See N. Kanellopoulou, "Reciprocity, trust, and public interest in research biobanking", p. 45-53.

Federal Ministry of Education and Research, the Austrian Federal Ministry of Science and Research and the Academy of Finland under grant number 01GP0905A.

Public Health – It Is Running Through My Veins: Personalized Medicine and Individual Responsibility for Health

Martin LANGANKE, Tobias FISCHER, Kyle B. BROTHERS

Abstract: This article critiques the thesis that Personalized Medicine will create a new culture of individual responsibility. Our main thesis is that the connection between PM and individual responsibility is not as obvious as often assumed. This connection will only be put into practice if PM can fulfill its scientific promise and specific political decisions are made. These political decisions are not given in the results of PM research. If "responsibility" is defined as a four-way relation, and basic health economics considerations are chosen as a set of rules, the following can be concluded: A necessary but not sufficient requirement is fulfilled if PM can show practical success in the prediction of diseases that are partly modifiable and partly constitutional. Beyond this requirement though, further policy changes with ethical, legal and political dimensions would need to be made in order for PM to provide a basis for a new kind of individual responsibility. These policy changes will need to account for the medical possibilities as well as the significant challenges inherent in practices such as sanctioning and monitoring behavior. It is apparent that a new understanding of individual responsibility can only enter practice if relevant political decisions are made and this is unlikely, because many of the required changes are highly questionable from a political and ethical point of view.

1 Introduction

Emerging fields of research within medicine have frequently raised questions concerning our conceptions of humankind and definitions of what it is to be human. At times they have even profoundly influenced our concepts of "personhood." Both the mechanistic model of the 17th century and the notion of "experimenting doctors" in the second half of the 19th century are examples of this phenomenon. Developments in the field of medicine have led to new heuristics, and research programs have advanced methods which have shaken the foundation of so-called "assured knowledge" about humankind.

149

Even now fields within health research carry the potential to influence our basic notions of anthropology, and a number of commentators have proposed that Personalized Medicine (PM) is one such field of research.[1] For these scholars, one source for the potential anthropological impact of the current discourse concerning PM lies in the way it can alter our understanding of health and sickness.[2]

PM is likely to influence our understanding in at least two ways. Firstly, PM has the potential to drive the construction of new anthropological categories such as the "healthy sick"[3] and the "sickly well." Secondly, PM has the potential to reframe "self-control" in regard to a patient's own health status. PM aims to enable patients to actively "manage" their own health and sickness, but at the same time this has the potential to intensify the focus on their responsibility for their own well-being.[4] In this second vision

---

[1] For further insight into the discussion concerning Personalized Medicine see O. Golubnitschaja (Ed.), *Predictive Diagnostics and Personalized Treatment: Dream or Reality*, New York 2009; R. Kollek, T. Lemke (Eds.), *Der medizinische Blick in die Zukunft. Gesellschaftliche Implikationen prädiktiver Gentests*, Frankfurt 2008; W. Niederlag, H. U. Lemke, O. Golubnitschaja, O. Rienhoff (Eds.), *Personalisierte Medizin*, Health Academy 14, Dresden 2010 as well as A. Smart, P. Martin, M. Parker, "Tailored Medicine: Whom will it fit? The ethics of patient and disease stratification", in: *Bioethics*, 18(4)/2004, p. 322-343. A good survey of the different approaches to PM is given by B. Hüsing, J. Hartig, B. Bührlen, T. Reiß, S. Gaisser (Eds.), *Individualisierte Medizin und Gesundheitssystem*, TAB-Arbeitsbericht 126, Berlin 2008. Aspects of research ethics within the context of Personalized Medicine are discussed by M. Langanke, K. B. Brothers, P. Erdmann, J. Weinert, J. Krfczyk-Korth, M. Dörr, W. Hoffmann, H. K. Krömer, H. Assel, "Comparing different scientific approaches to Personalized Medicine: research ethics and privacy protection", in: *Personalized Medicine*, 8(4)/2011, p. 437-444.

[2] For a survey of both terms see: A. Franke, *Modelle von Gesundheit und Krankheit. Lehrbuch Gesundheitswissenschaften*, Bern 2010; M. Gadebusch Bondio, S. Michl, "Die neue Medizin und ihre Versprechen", in: *Deutsches Ärzteblatt*, 107(21)/2010, A-1062, B-934, C-922.

[3] Exemplary of this strand of discussion: H. Kamps, "Deutsches Gesundheitswesen: Gut für die gesunden Kranken", in: *Deutsches Ärzteblatt*, 105(23)/2008, A-1276, B-1105, C-1081; M. Myrtek, *Gesunde Kranke, kranke Gesunde*, Bern 1998.

[4] See D. Schäfer, A. Frewer, E. Schockenhoff, V. Wetzstein (Eds.), *Gesundheitskonzepte im Wandel. Geschichte, Ethik und Gesellschaft*, Geschichte und Philosophie der Medizin 6, Stuttgart 2008; M. Rothhaar, A. Frewer (Eds.), *Das Gesunde, das Kranke und die Medizintechnik. Moralische Implikationen des Krankheitsbegriffs*, Geschichte und Philosophie der Medizin 12, Stuttgart 2012.

of the future, "health" and "sickness" could be moved permanently from the sphere of the naturally occurring to the domain of the technically and culturally determined.

Expectations about how patients can control their health through PM have been examined in the fields of politics, medicine, and scientific studies. Ulla Burchardt, chair of the committee for Education and Research of the German Bundestag, has argued that PM depends on responsible citizens and patients who are willing and able to participate and change their attitudes.[5] In reference to this comment, Bärbel Hüsing, author of the 2008 study "Individualisierte Medizin und Gesundheitssystem" concludes that "Personalized Medicine is often argumentatively linked to individual responsibility."[6]

Following the point of view of Regine Kollek, PM should be understood as a health-scientific approach that enables as well as obligates patients and recipients of benefits to maintain or reconstitute their own health. "Personalized Medicine will change the assumption that health and illness are solely affected by chance and fate, but rather that they are the object and result of will. 'If health is the result of will, illness must be a side effect of a missing or misguided will,'" says Kollek.[7]

Although these three statements emphasize different elements of the issue, they all agree on the correlation between the promises made by PM and the capacity of every person to maintain or re-establish his or her own health. These approaches all refer to the problem of *individual responsibility*. It seems that within the framework of the potential that advocates claim for PM, chance and risk in relation to PM are indelibly linked to the issue of individual responsibility. While it is difficult to speak of PM as if it is a well-defined field of research with a clear core of theoretical assumptions, goals, and research methods, the biomarker-based approach is a particularly well-defined field of research within PM. Biomarker-based Personalized Medicine (bPM) raises questions about the management of risk which are directly linked to the issue of individual responsibility for health.

5   U. Hempel, "Personalisierte Medizin I, Keine Heilkunst mehr, sondern rationale molekulare Wissenschaft", in: *Deutsches Ärzteblatt,* 106(42)/2009,A-2068, B-1769, C-1733, A-2068.
6   U. Hempel, "Personalisierte Medizin I", A-2070.
7   U. Hempel, "Personalisierte Medizin I", A-2070.

We will examine how these questions are raised by the biomarker approach in order to point to the central role this issue plays in PM in general.

2 Personalized Medicine as Predictive Medicine – the Biomarker-Based Approach

Biomarker-based Personalized Medicine centers on the practice of using values acquired through specialized laboratory tests to estimate the probability that certain clinical events will occur for a particular patient. These laboratory values, called biomarkers, might be used to estimate the probability that a patient will respond or fail to respond to a treatment or whether they will develop a particular disease. Alternatively, they can create a personal risk profile for a range of possible events. In some cases a single biomarker is used, but a combination of biomarkers may be required to derive accurate estimates.

Initially, the term "biomarker" was used exclusively to refer to genetic markers, especially single nucleotide polymorphisms (SNPs). More recently, biomarker research has come to include a range of potential laboratory values. The project "Greifswald Approach to Individualized Medicine" (GANI_MED) carried out by the University of Greifswald is an example of a research project focused on a wide range of biomarkers. This project involves researchers looking for biomarkers across a range of "Omics" fields, including genomics, transcriptomics, proteomics, and metabolomics. Despite the use of emerging areas of biomedical research, bPM in general, and the GANI_MED project in particular, retain essentially the same focus as classic tools of early detection. The goal is to initiate measures that can minimize morbidity from certain diseases and significantly improve the effectiveness of therapies. bPM is an advance over previous early detection methods primarily in its focus on detecting disease risk before the patient has become ill or, once a disease has developed, to select the treatment option that is most likely to be successful for an individual patient.

It is apparent from this that the term "biomarker" applies not only to laboratory values that are used to identify the personal risk of a patient to develop an illness, but also tests intended to improve the chance of success in treatment. This article will focus on the elements of biomarker-based Personalized Medicine that relate to disease prediction. Our aim is to explicate the connections between bPM and individual responsibility, and it is this connection which carries the potential to influence conceptions of anthropology. In light of this goal, we will exclude biomarker-based predictions aimed at improving the success of therapies, since the dimensions of individual responsibility we will be concerned with here are raised most acutely in cases where a person is expected to prevent themselves from developing a disease or diseases.

3 PM and Responsibility – Preliminary Considerations

We will argue that, based on the framing for biomarker research introduced above, a new form of individual responsibility is constructed through the use of biomarkers to predict the development of disease. While on the one hand biomarkers are intended to be used to present information on the predisposition of apparently healthy persons to develop diseases, many of the diseases that are particularly well suited for prediction through bPM are currently considered to be avoidable through lifestyle change. Management of some of these diseases already involves clinical risk tools, such as risk algorithms for myocardial infarction. In the scenario created by bPM, a patient identified to be at an increased risk for developing a disease is simultaneously empowered and obligated to manage their own risk for developing that disease.

Depending on the political and social context, this scenario could take the form of either a medical promise of salvation or a catastrophe. From an optimistic point of view, bPM could enable well-informed individuals to improve or modify their lifestyle in a way that is guided by their personal risk. Through the use of this approach, common preventable threats to health might be mitigated or even eliminated. But negative implications can also be expected. Among these implications are (1) a shift of responsibility for health from medical providers to the patient, (2) the limitation of benefits to those patients who are well-informed and educated and thus able to understand and interpret risk productively, and (3) further exacerbation of a loss of solidarity in public health care systems. Solidarity is potentially at risk, because a shift of responsibility towards patients creates an environment where sanctions, including financial sanctions, could be applied to patients who fail to change health behaviors.

This issue is having a significant influence on the public discourse in Germany. German health care is financed primarily through a socialized system, so concern about solidarity within the health care system is of greater urgency than it is, for example, in the United States, where the health care system is driven predominantly by the private sector. For this reason, Personalized Medicine is a topic of great importance in the political debate around health in this country. That Personalized Medicine carries such a political charge in the German context further justifies engaging a deeper examination of the relationships between Personalized Medicine and individual responsibility for health. More precisely, in relation to the public discourse in Germany, it will be essential to examine individual responsibility in light of the promises made by bPM in order to identify, as accurately as possible, to what extent and under which premises bPM is a driver of changes in claims about the way individuals can and should take charge of their health. This article will seek to clarify this issue in four steps: First, we will analyze the concept of "individual responsibility" in terms of its logical and paradigmatic implications. Secondly, we will clarify the term "individual responsibility" logically and semantically with respect to the specific context of health. Thirdly, we will propose the features that bPM must have in order for us to meaningfully discuss how it might impose a new kind of individual responsibility for health on patients. Finally, we will clarify the issues outside of medicine that could potentially transform a conceptual shift in the concept of individual responsibility into significant changes in the delivery of health care.

4 Logical and pragmatic implications of "responsibility"

Even before the topic of Personalized Medicine came to the fore, there was already a public discourse about the issue of individual responsibility with respect to socialized public health care systems. The question of whether or not individuals are responsible in the maintenance and restoration of their own health has been addressed in other settings; it has even been considered by law. In the fifth book of the German Social Security Code (Sozialgeset-zbuch V) the first paragraph states (§1, solidarity and individual responsibility): "Insured persons are *jointly responsible* for their health; they should contribute to their health by means of a health-conscious lifestyle, early involvement in preventive health measures, and through active participation in medical treatment and rehabilitation, in order to prevent the development of disease and disability or to prevent the consequences of disease and disability" (emphasis added, translation by authors).

Although the German Social Security Code mentions the concept of self-responsibility or co-responsibility as an integral part of the socialized health insurance system, these receive no further comment and are not defined. The use of this term in the German Social Security Code appears to rely on a definition that is in common usage.

A variety of meanings are associated with the term responsibility, depending on the context. It seems that one meaning for this term is used informally in a wide range of contexts. In this common usage, responsibility refers to the demand on a person or an institution to justify its action towards another person or institution. It is worth noting that this requirement for justification emerges only in settings where the compliance of the person or institution with the relevant rules or requirements is under question. This preliminary understanding of responsibility can be understood as a relation among four variables:[8]

W is responsible to Y for X because of certain normative standard Z.[9]

Within this equation W and Y are placeholders for individuals or institutions. X stands for an action or an omission. Z stands for particular norms, including commandments, prohibitions, permissions, or even a larger normative system.

In this definition of responsibility, action as well as omission may need to be justified.[10] It does not make sense to demand the assumption of responsibility for an act that has no element of omission or commission, since

---

[8]   See G. Marckmann, M. Möhrle, A. Blum, "Gesundheitliche Eigenverantwortung. Möglichkeiten und Grenzen am Beispiel des malignen Melanoms.", in: *Der Hautarzt*, 55/2004, p. 715-720, p. 716.

[9]   For this formulation see also M. H. Werner, "Verantwortung", in: ders., M. Düwell, C. Hübenthal (Eds.), *Handbuch Ethik*, ³Stuttgart 2011, p. 541-548; as well as R. Hillerbrandt (Ed.), *Technik, Ökologie, Ethik. Ein normativer Grundlagendiskurs über den Umgang mit Wissenschaft, Technik und Umwelt*, Paderborn 2006, p. 36 f. Much more complex formulations for the relationships relevant to responsibility may be found, including some with six or seven elements.

[10] See also G. Marckmann et al., "Gesundheitliche Eigenverantwortung", p. 715-720.

responsibility relates to the effect on the other person or institution that is caused by the action. The concept of responsibility is therefore connected inextricably with the concepts of action and omission (or "negative" action); this connection has several consequences that are pertinent to this discussion:

a) An individual or institution is only responsible for an action with respect to the consequences of that action. This is the case if an event or situation can be understood as being caused by the action, and if the event or situation can be judged to be desirable or undesirable (i.e. not neutral) with respect to the rules or values in a certain setting.

b) It follows from this first consequence that if it is uncertain which out of two potential acts caused a desirable or undesirable situation to develop, it will necessarily be problematic to claim or attribute responsibility with respect to either act.

Responsibility concerning a certain action can be understood retrospectively as well as prospectively. It is possible to distinguish between responsibility of competence and responsibility of accountability.[11]

a) Responsibility of competence (prospective): An individual or an institution bears responsibility for something which must be rendered in the future.

b) Responsibility of accountability (retrospective): An individual or institution is held responsible – *after the event* – for the results or consequences which have already occurred as a result of an action performed by that individual or institution.

In light of this distinction between responsibility of competence and of accountability, we can see that a relationship exists between the two forms of responsibility: "Only if someone, on the basis of normative standards, bears prospective responsibility for a situation can he then be held retrospectively accountable if he has not fulfilled this obligation in accordance with the prescribed standard."[12]

Going further, there are three aspects of an action that are necessary to claim

---

[11] For the following see G. Marckmann et al., "Gesundheitliche Eigenverantwortung", p. 715-720; G. Marckmann, "Präventionsmaßnahmen im Spannungsfeld zwischen individueller Autonomie und allgemeinem Wohl", in: *Ethik in der Medizin,* 22(3)/2010, p. 207-220.

[12] G. Marckmann et al., "Gesundheitliche Eigenverantwortung", p. 716.

or attribute responsibility with respect to a resulting situation:

a) Self-dependence: An action needs to be performed with minimal coercion in order for responsibility to be attributed to the agent, otherwise responsibility is shifted from the coerced agent towards the coercing individual or institution.

b) Availability of alternative actions: If someone is held accountable for an action, a feasible alternative action needs to have been available. Responsibility reaches its logical limit if the possibility to act otherwise neither existed nor exists.

c) Level of information: To hold an agent accountable for an action, prospectively as well as retrospectively, that agent needs to have known the possible results of both the action and the alternative actions, or at least *should* have known the possible results. "Responsibility" within the medical context

Having defined responsibility in this way, we now need to turn to the task of identifying how responsibility can be defined within the general context of medical care. We take the idea of responsibility for one's own health to mean that one's health is the object of one's own responsibility.[13]

4.1 Illness as the object of responsibility

Following on from the above discussion on the relationship between action and responsibility, we can see that personal health status may be an object of responsibility, if it can be modified through action on the part of the individual. Many diseases are candidates for being objects of responsibility because their development or course is considered to be influenced by personal lifestyle. This includes illnesses that can be prevented through physical activity and healthy nutrition, as well as illnesses whose development is affected by certain behaviors, such as smoking tobacco. In addition, diseases could be regarded as the responsibility of the patient even though they are not affected by lifestyle or health behaviors, such as those whose course and severity is modifiable by screenings and preventive health assessments.

---

[13] Alternatively, individual responsibility could be defined as a responsibility in which the object and the authority of responsibility are the same. In this article this definition is not used.

Certain types of cancer would fit this category, since their prognosis may be improved by an early diagnosis.

The potential for individual responsibility does not extend to all diseases, however, since some diseases cannot, according to current knowledge, be modified through the action of the individual, and must therefore be treated as an unfortunate situation which occurs through no action or inaction on the part of the patient.[14] Conditions of this type include those which are determined exclusively through genetic causes, or can be traced back to given environmental conditions or unavoidable working conditions. The phenomenon of addiction, among other medico-social phenomena, presents problems of various kinds within this scheme.

Individual responsibility in the medical context can also be construed prospectively and retrospectively. A patient who has developed a disease as a result of unhealthy behaviors could be held responsible retrospectively once treatment for that disease begins to require medical resources beyond those that would have been needed had he or she not engaged in healthy behaviors. Likewise, an individual could be held responsible prospectively for an unhealthy lifestyle, since that lifestyle could lead to the development of diseases which require treatments.

A special consideration applies, however, to prospective responsibility. Since we regard persons to be responsible for their behaviors only if they could have chosen otherwise (recall our observation about coercion), then prospective responsibility is indelibly linked to access to relevant information. Only if someone is informed about health risks which result from a certain lifestyle, as well as alternative behaviors that might be pursued, can he or she choose not to engage in the relevant health behaviors. This has been called the "criterion of the level of information."[15] Undoubtedly, only if a patient has had access to adequate information could he or she become subject to a penalty or other forms of responsibility for failing to avoid a

---

[14] For a discussion on "to befall" see W. Kamlah, *Philosophische Anthropologie, Sprachkritische Grundlegung und Ethik*, Mannheim/Wien/Zürich 1972, p. 34-40 and B. Marx (Ed.), *Widerfahrnis und Erkenntnis: Zur Wahrheit menschlicher Erfahrung*, Leipzig 2010.

[15] See N. Paul, "Medizinische Prädiktion, Prävention und Gerechtigkeit: Anmerkungen zu ethischen Dimensionen eines biomedizinischen Ideals", in: *Ethik in der Medizin*, 22(3)/2010, p. 191-205, p. 197.

risk behavior or take preventive measures.

Going further, all the criteria for responsibility noted above remain valid even in the context of a public health system built on the concept of joint responsibility.[16] It is clear that joint responsibility is a more useful concept than exclusive responsibility in the realm of health and health care. This is because there are virtually no diseases that develop in individuals exclusively as a result of their own avoidable behaviors and actions. Notwithstanding a range of political ideologies presenting extremist views, health risks are virtually always the result of combinations of factors that can be controlled by individuals, such as health behaviors and utilization of preventive measures, and those that are beyond the control of individuals, such as genetic and environmental factors.[17] There are very few phenomena in human health that can be attributed in a straightforward way to a single cause, and only a few more that can be attributed to multiple factors that are all controllable. Since this is the case, it is only possible to connect responsibility to those elements of risk that are regarded to be modifiable. However, even within this limited scope the logical implications of responsibility still apply.

Similarly, joint responsibility with respect to recovery from illness is constrained by the responsibility of healthcare providers. This is not based on a traditional, paternalistic perspective on health care, but rather on the observation that it is necessary for a medical lay person to trust that the abilities of healthcare providers, as well as the therapeutic technologies they use, will bring about a return to health with minimal adverse effects. In this case, the patient is only responsible for those adverse effects of medical treatment that he or she could have deliberately modified. In such a scenario only the degree of the responsibility is limited. But the fundamental logical justification for the relevance of responsibility, as explained in section four, remains unaffected.

---

[16] See T. Krpić –Močilar, *Mitverantwortung für die eigene Gesundheit*. Studien zur Rechtswissenschaft 122, Hamburg 2003.

[17] M. Düngen, "Genetische Disposition und medizinische Behandlung"; http://www.bpb. de/themen/J6B7SV,1,0,Genetische_Disposition_und_medizinische_Behandlung.html.

4.2 Authority of responsibility and the rules of a socialized health care system

We need to address two additional issues in relation to the attribution of responsibility within the medical context – issues which arise in light of the relation between responsibility and the relevant system of rules.

Authority of Responsibility

As noted above, responsibility depends on some authority, since without authority responsibility would create no obligation. What kind of authority applies to the context of medical treatments? This question is not addressed in the statements quoted earlier from the German Social Security Code. An obvious assumption could be that the insured person is responsible to the community of insured persons, or perhaps an institution which represents their interests. If this is the case, then the responsibility could be understood in the following way: Every member of the compulsory health insurance system in Germany pays a certain fee to a common fund. This fund is used to pay for medical treatments that are covered through this arrangement. The rules and standards can be changed over time as a result of changes in the state of medical knowledge, but at any point in time it is relatively clear which costs are covered, and at what rate. It is presumed that the costs of medications with uncertain effectiveness, as well as treatments which are selected on the basis of personal taste rather than medical evidence are not covered by the insurance fund. Based on this framework, it is in the interest of all members of such an insurance community to maintain enough available funds to cover the costs of every treatment which members need. If the financial resources of the fund are limited, and if the fees paid by the members cannot be increased enough to maintain solvency, problems develop. In this way, it is questionable whether treatments of diseases which can be avoided by the patient should be paid. An even more serious problem arises if, through the coverage of treatments of diseases that could have been avoided, the quality and the quantity of other benefits are diminished.

The first paragraph of the fifth book of the German Social Security Code can be seen as a plea to insured persons to look after their own health status as much as they can, in order to control costs and avoid higher fees or reduced benefits. Such a demand may seem appropriate in Germany in light of its socialized health care system and aging society.

It can therefore be said that the insured individual can be held responsible for their own health with respect to the community of insured people and the compulsory health insurance fund. It remains questionable which sanctioning mechanisms the institution representing the community of insured people should possess. It is clear that such a mechanism would need to possess certain powers in order to enforce the responsibility for health. These powers should enable the authority to sanction an undesired unhealthy behavior, or to encourage the adoption of healthier behaviors. If it is agreed that an institution possesses the authority to sanction certain actions, three challenges become apparent:

– Are only positive sanctions accepted, that is the encouragement of good behavior through bonuses; or are negative sanctions, such as increasing fees for those non-compliant with rules, also warranted?
– Which actions or lifestyle choices need to be sanctioned and by what criteria?
– How should the institution determine whether a behavior susceptible to sanction has been committed? To formulate the problem more acutely: Should the authority be able to verify if a person quit smoking or at least reduced his or her use? Is a voluntary disclosure of the insured individual sufficient? How extensive can such an investigative power be?

System of Rules

The fifth book of the German Social Security Code provides no system of rules to define the responsibilities it attributes to citizens/patients. Without a set of rules and interdictions, though, it is impossible to distinguish between behavior which is considered responsible, or perhaps *compliant*, and behavior which conflicts with the rules. But the ability to make such judgments about behaviors is a necessary prerequisite to apply a system of reward or sanction. Following the construct of responsibility drawn by the German Social Security Code, what kind of behavior is obligatory for the insured person and what actions or omissions are considered to be violations of the rules?

The concept of solidarity may provide some normative guidance for such a set of guidelines. Some work has already been undertaken to frame individual responsibility for health in terms of solidarity.[18] From our point of view, the following two suggestions provide a starting point for enacting the concept of solidarity into a system capable of assessing behavior in the context of a compulsory health insurance system.

a) The precept of thriftiness: The community of members of the compulsory health insurance fund share an interest in ensuring that the fund exercises thrift in the use of available resources. Preventable costs should be avoided. This does not solely affect the administration of the fund itself, but also the reimbursement of expenses. The costs of treatments deriving from diseases that are considered avoidable provide a possible avenue for sanction. For example, a smoker may be held responsible for the cost of diseases resulting from their cigarette consumption. We can envision an approach in which a list of diseases is published that categorizes conditions as avoidable or unavoidable according to current medical knowledge. Reimbursement for costs resulting from these diseases could then be withheld, or only partial reimbursement might be provided.

b) Interdiction against the misuse of resources: The compulsory health insurance system could alternatively set up a system to prevent the misuse of resources. Resources could be understood as misused if they are spent on treatments for avoidable diseases. Implemented through a list of diseases resulting from unhealthy behaviors, patients could be held responsible and sanctioned for avoidable use of resources.

The choice to place authority to set and administer such rules with the compulsory health insurance, rather than its members, might raise some discomfort. But in this conception the health insurance system is understood as an institutional representative of the interests of its members. Therefore, these two normative rules can be rephrased and can even be combined into one rule: "All members of a health-care system organized socially are

---

[18] See Marckmann et al., "Gesundheitliche Eigenverantwortung"; M. Rohr, D. Schade, *Selbstbestimmung und Eigenverantwortung im Gesundheitswesen – Ergebnisse des Workshops zu Forschungsbedarf im Bereich Medizin und Gesundheit*. Akademie für Technikfolgenabschätzung in Baden-Württemberg, Arbeitsbericht Nr. 176, Stuttgart 2000.

obliged to prevent costs of treatments for avoidable diseases, and in this respect make as thrifty and non-abusive use of resources as possible."

5 PM – A tool for the self-management of health?

We have demonstrated so far that the challenges that arise in relation to individual responsibility in the context of health are apparent even without reference to biomarker-based Personalized Medicine. bPM is an emerging approach to health that even when successful, will be confronted with several of the problems discussed above. As medicine begins to utilize these novel methods for the precise prediction of diseases, the discourse on individual responsibility will be brought to the fore. If this matter is analyzed accurately, the following becomes obvious: bPM is a tool that could change the conception of individual responsibility. This change might render responsibility more transparent, but it could also make it more demanding. In the following, we will discuss some of the necessary but not yet sufficient prerequisites for establishing a relationship between Personalized Medicine and individual responsibility. These criteria will need to be met in order for individual responsibility for health to take a more significant role in the health care system through bPM.

Bearing in mind that we have so far argued that:

a) The attribution of responsibility in a medical context requires that it is possible for the object of responsibility to be directly influenced by the responsible person.

b) Let us consider a situation where action A is linked to result Z, and action B is an alternative to action A. If it is uncertain that pursuing action B can prevent result Z, it is questionable whether the choice to continue to pursue action A needs to be justified.

c) In order to hold an agent responsible, it has to be presupposed that they were aware of the alternative actions available as well as of all of the potential effects.

Only actions and their effects need to be considered to fall into the domain of responsibility. This basic supposition does not easily apply in the context of bPM. The prerequisite that a disease or condition must be considered to be avoidable or modifiable does not seem to apply in the fields of bPM related to genetic markers or diseases for which people are genetically pre-disposed. If bPM only enhances predictive knowledge through genetic risk profiles and does not provide options for individual or medical interventions to alter this risk, then little benefit will be provided to patients. However, if bPM is used as a predictive tool to improve the management of conditions that are susceptible to intervention, then bPM may support the attribution of individual responsibility. Under these circumstances, bPM may open up possibilities for improved predictive and preventive health programs that target individual patient risks and might therefore provide more efficient care. We can see that such programs would fit into the category of "joint responsibility." Obviously the connection between bPM and individual re-sponsibility only works with those diseases which are, in regard to their occurrence and severity, the result of risks that are partly constitutional and partly modifiable. And it is inherent in the definition of biomarkers that they reflect a physiology that is at least partly constitutional. Thus, responsibil-ity only applies to those diseases which can also be modified by lifestyle or behavior changes. This requirement is only fulfilled for those diseases where the genetic predisposition to develop the disease can be triggered by behavior or environmental conditions. In the context of such diseases only a joint responsibility can be logically assumed.

Joint responsibility relates not only to the limited modifiability of dis-eases, but also to the limitations of responsibility introduced by the re-sponsibility of medical staff. It is expected that bPM will not create com-pletely new preventive programs, but will rather provide biomarker-based risk profiles to improve existing preventive programs. These profiles may guide the implementation of lifestyle changes or participation in preven-tion or surveillance-based programs. Taking obesity as an example, bPM may make it possible to distinguish between the so-called "metabolically healthy" obese and obesity that will lead to an increased risk for health conditions such as cardiovascular disease. This may result in healthcare providers providing advice to make lifestyle changes, but this advice will often only represent the strengthening of a medical advice which is routine for all patients. Since the practice of making health recommendations in-volves the timely and convincing efforts of healthcare providers, we can see that this is one way that patient's individual responsibility and the respon-sibility of the healthcare providers can come to overlap.

Let us return to the issue of minimal constraints on responsibility and their implication for the theory of action: A risk profile cannot be considered modifiable if the alternative action, i.e. a modification of lifestyle, does not carry with it a significant or reliable improvement in the risk or severity of the related disease. If a lifestyle change would only result in a minimal decrease in the risk to develop a disease, it is not evident that an adherence to the current lifestyle violates, for example, the precept of thriftiness. On the other hand, a violation against the precept of thriftiness within a set of rules can only be sanctioned if the adherence to current lifestyle implies a significantly higher risk to become ill.

bPM can only strengthen individual responsibility if it can be shown that changes in lifestyle or participation in preventive programs are linked to a significantly decreased risk for developing conditions or a decreased severity of diseases once they have developed. Furthermore, the results of bPM will only affect individual responsibility if the proper lab tests are performed and the results are made available to patients along with a clear explanation of their significance. As mentioned earlier, the availability of an adequate amount of information is a necessary constraint to the application of individual responsibility in a medical context. If the connection between health behaviors and their consequences is unknown, then it cannot be expected that changes will be made.

As we have said, it is possible that bPM will guide not only basic health advice ("Eat more fruit and vegetables, exercise, and quit drinking"), but also new preventive strategies for certain diseases. The success of both of these avenues will depend in part on public health communication efforts. Even though healthcare providers will be able to order the right tests, interpret the results, and work with patients to respond properly, the availability of such interventions would need to be widely known in order for citizens to be held responsible in case of non-compliance.

In addition to the considerations that arise from responsibility, as we have discussed above, two issues particularly relevant to bPM need to be discussed further:

a) It is clear that the accuracy of risk estimates for the development of disease available through bPM will vary widely. Only if estimates have a high level of sensitivity and specificity can claims to individual responsibility hold sway.[19] Findings for which there is only weak evidence to support a correlation do not rise to the level of affirmatively demanding action on the part of the patient.

b) Assuming that a financial set of rules underlie the issue of individual responsibility for health in the context of a socialized health care system has significant implications for the system as a whole. To reframe healthcare as a primarily utilitarian endeavor, as the precept of thriftiness and the interdiction against the misuse of resources seem to do, is also to demand that the system as a whole follow these rules. To study a rare type of cancer with "omics"-related methods may be justified in the context of basic or clinical research, but not by economic arguments. Even if it becomes possible for advances related to such rare conditions to be translated into clinical care in a way that both mortality and treatment expenses are lowered, the overall financial benefit to the healthcare system will be small. Advances in science related to bPM and changes in clinical care guided by it might be required to reduce the cost of treatments. The healthcare system might even require that bPM efforts focus on diseases the treatments of which produce the highest costs.

6 Non-medical frameworks – the normative level

Even if we conclude that applications of bPM meet the logical prerequisites for creating individual responsibilities, we need not conclude that sanctions are the appropriate mechanism for translating that responsibility into policy. The implementation of policies falls within the domain of politics, and

---

[19] If the specificity of a biomarker is understood as the ability to identify those at low-risk for developing disease with a high statistical accuracy, the following can be stated: The more the specificity of a biomarker decreases, the greater the number of false positive predictions it produces. A biomarker, which is in this sense non-specific, is unable to serve as the basis for individual responsibility in a clinical context. This reasoning applies for sensitivity in an analogical way. If the sensitivity of a biomarker is understood as the ability to identify accurately those at increased risk, the following can be claimed: the more the sensitivity of a biomarker decreases, the greater the number of false negative predictions it produces. For tests with low specificity, the result of a biomarker-based test could easily be treated as a "false alarm," and in this case a decision not to change one's lifestyle would not be unreasonable.

is therefore debatable by normative standards. In fact, the implementation of policies related to individual responsibility in a compulsory health insurance system would require changes in the "contract" that governs the relationships of citizens to the system and to one another. Such changes would require a normative justification.

The logical connections between PM and individual responsibility for health might suggest that medical innovations related to bPM will automatically lead to changes in the policies of a health care system related to individual responsibility. This expectation was expressed by Bärbel Hüsing in the quote provided above. But we find this expectation to be flawed.

Research on bPM may succeed in identifying biomarkers that can identify disease risks with a high sensitivity and specificity. But it is questionable whether patients belonging to such risk groups can be held responsible if they act in a way that is different from that which is medically advised. This is true, in part, because the implementation of policies that link personal responsibility with biomarker-based interventions in a socialized health care system is an extremely complex challenge. Many steps would be needed for such a change, and these steps involve considerations that extend beyond the scientific/clinical scope.

The following questions mark issues that would need to be considered in any policy changes that enact personal responsibility into a socialized healthcare system:

a) Which disease risks amenable to biomarker-based prediction and modification through health behaviors should be included into the group of illnesses susceptible to sanction?

b) Which tests should be authorized for implementation into the medical routine in order to identify certain markers? Will the costs of these tests be covered by the compulsory health insurance system?

c) Should participation in biomarker-based screening be compulsory for diseases which are defined as subject to sanction?

d) Which preventive or predictive programs should a person who has been identified as at risk through a biomarker-based test be required to attend? Are those expenses covered?

e) How will an adequate level of information be delivered to the public? Which tasks arise for physicians in private practice?

f) How can and should the institution check whether a behavior in need of sanction is taking place?

g) Finally, which sanctions are acceptable? This affects the regulations concerning *c.* and the issue of behavior and lifestyle mentioned in *f*. Both a reward and a punishment system could be implemented.

In listing these issues within political and normative dimensions, it becomes clear that some changes would be more difficult to implement than others. However, some of these issues have already been addressed in other medical settings. For example, licensure of tests could help address issue *b* noted above. An example of this process is the licensure of the pharmacogenomic test which can be used to determine the likelihood of the success of Herceptin, a therapy for breast cancer patients.[20] Although the level of standardization for this laboratory test may be criticized, the Herceptin test is a good example how a licensure can improve patient-centered care.

The implementation of screening programs as mentioned in *d* is already used in practice, too. An example for this would be the breast cancer screenings which are most widely offered in Germany. These screenings are offered by the insurance program for women starting at a certain age. However, we are not aware of any proposals for the costs of breast cancer treatment to be dependent on participation in screenings, especially among high risk patients. Nevertheless, the example of breast cancer screenings shows that preventive screenings can be offered for the vast majority of members of the general public.

If necessary, a large-scale public education program including physicians in private practice could be carried out in order to achieve a higher level of information for the general public. The health insurance system already uses information letters to brief patients, and these are targeted according to patients' risks. Such communication methods could be used to inform insured citizens about biomarker-based screenings and preventive programs.

It is not inevitable that the creation of a list, as anticipated in *a*, would fail because of insuperable problems. If the political will to radically recon-

---

[20] For information on Herceptin therapy see: U. Hasler-Strub, "Aktuelle Therapien beim metastasierten Brustkrebs. Eine Übersicht über evidenzbasierte Optionen", in: *Schweizer Zeitschrift für Onkologie,* 5/2009, p. 20-22. Or visit: http://www.krebsinformationsdienst.de/tumorarten/brustkrebs/moderne-verfahren.php.

struct the public health care system is present, it might be possible to define which modifiable diseases are the targets of sanctions in case lifestyle or behavior changes are not adopted. This can be carried out through the guidance of the current state of medical knowledge and information about healthcare expenses. If biomedical research establishes a connection between lifestyle and the risk for contracting a disease, i.e. by statistical means, this assumption would be enough to implement a financial incentive, a positive sanction so to speak. The list which would be generated according to a, would need to be revised frequently depending on the current state of medical knowledge. If opinions concerning these diseases change, a revision of the list would become necessary.

While solutions to some of the problems, which are linked to the points a, b, d and e, do exist, the implementation of policies related to the issues raised in the points c, f and g would lead to severe limitations on the rights of insured persons.

Regarding c: The question of whether risk screenings should be obligatory is controversial, particularly in the context of so called "public health genomics." In Germany this debate was strongly influenced by Peter Dabrock; his clear yet provocative position states that participation in risk-screenings which fulfill certain procedural and ethical presumptions is ethically more justifiable than refusal. In this case it cannot be ruled out that under certain circumstances participation in screenings may be obligatory.[21]

Dabrock's theses can be characterized as fundamental socio-ethical assumptions. Moreover, they indicate that the scenario to make certain screenings obligatory is not completely rejected by the community of ethicists, who act as consultants in political decisions about health and social issues. We will not address here the question of whether such reasoning is sustainable. For this article it is only important to show that a course of action such as the one mentioned in c is an explosive issue. It would be a misuse of the conception of bPM to state that something inherent in PM can be used to decide anything concerning the implementation of obligatory screenings. It is the task of democratically-authorized policy-making bodies to decide whether policy changes should be based on the interpretation

---

[21]   See P. Dabrock, "Public Health Genetics and Social Justice", in: *Community Genetics*, 9(1)/2006, p. 34-39.

of political and ethical issues. In other words, these are normative issues, not purely scientific ones. Decisions cannot be made on the basis of evidence that bPM can show successes in modifying disease risk or course. The fact that such medical benefits can be provided for patients does not automatically lead to the conclusion that all patients should engage in the necessary interventions.

The same arguments apply by analogy to the issue raised in f. If a political will to implement monitoring of health behaviors does in fact develop, numerous instruments of control could be adopted. One example is the introduction of certificates which attest participation in early diagnostics or in consultations to change lifestyle accordingly. Such mechanisms are now used within the health care system in the form of bonus cards. This could be seen as an obvious, if positive, sanctioning mechanism. An alternative could be a process in which the insured patient is obliged to truthfully provide information about his or her own lifestyle if costs for treatments of preventable diseases occur. A similar procedure is used at the initiation of private health or life insurance policies. A third possibility is the use of laboratory tests to reliably evaluate certain behaviors.[22] This last option would represent an extreme move. Before such "lifestyle-tests" can be implemented in widespread practice, and before the results could be connected with sanctions, a drastic change in the political climate would need to occur.

Concerning the question of the nature of sanctions raised in g, it would be necessary to determine whether partly modifiable diseases are included in the list of diseases susceptible to sanction. If, as a justification of negative sanctions, they were to require a patient to contribute to his or her own costs, this would not be trivial. If a disease is considered to be avoidable by 80%, should the insured individual cover 80% of the costs if the disease occurs and relevant behavior changes have not been adopted? Something similar is done in legal practice in relation to the assignment of procedural costs. Yet, by choosing such a mechanism, the system would be strongly

---

[22] Advances in the field of Personalized Medicine itself would complicate the use of such tests. See for example, G. E. Swan, C. N. Lessov-Schlaggar, A. W. Bergen, Y. He, R. F. Tyndale, N. L. Benowitz, "Genetic and environmental influences on the ratio of 3'hydroxycotinine to cotinine in plasma and urine", in: *Pharmacogenetics,* 19(5)/2009, p. 388-398.

dependent on the current state of research, and therefore, would be under constant change. And this is not even to speak of the persistent scientific disagreement concerning the relative benefit of such health behaviors.

7 Conclusion

We have argued that there is a need to critically consider the thesis that Personalized Medicine will create a new culture of individual responsibility. The connection between PM and individual responsibility is not as obvious as initially presumed. The connection only exists if PM can fulfill its promise and political decisions – wanted or unwanted – are made, decisions which are not automatically given in the results of PM research. If "responsibility" is defined as a four-way relation and basic health economic considerations are chosen as a set of rules, the following can be concluded: A necessary but not sufficient requirement is fulfilled if bPM can show practical success in the prediction of diseases that are partly modifiable and partly constitutional. Beyond this requirement, though, further policy changes with ethical, legal and political dimensions would need to be made in order for PM to provide a basis for a new kind of individual responsibility. Those policy changes will need to account for the medical possibilities, as well as the significant challenges inherent in practices such as sanctioning and monitoring behavior. It is apparent that a new understanding of individual responsibility can only enter practice if relevant political decisions are made. Many of these required changes are highly questionable from a political and ethical point of view. The following issues may be the most controversial ones:
– Should participation in screenings be obligatory?
– Should compliance with medically-indicated health behaviors be monitored?
– Should negative sanctions, i.e. personal contributions to treatment costs, be implemented? Does this apply also to partly modifiable diseases? How can policies related to partly modifiable diseases be organized in a way that is practical without being arbitrary?
It is not the intent of this article to answer these ethical and politically explosive questions. In light of the aim of this publication, it is sufficient to state that those answers will not be given by PM itself. This validates

the thesis that PM cannot be the reason for a drastic reconstruction of the socially-financed public health care system. PM urges nobody to implement sanctions into the health care system. If such considerations are made, they have to be ethically, legally, and politically, i.e. normatively, justified. The political latitude to implement individual responsibility into the health care system is not affected by the advancement of scientific knowledge in the field of PM. In short, political discretion to develop the health care system cannot be restricted by arguments that attempt to eliminate the distinction between the way things are and the way things should be, not even in the setting of Personalized Medicine.

Acknowledgments

This work is part of the research project Greifswald Approach to Individualized Medicine (GANI_MED). The GANI_MED consortium is funded by the Federal Ministry of Education and Research and the Ministry of Cultural Affairs of the Federal State of Mecklenburg-West Pomerania (support codes: 03IS2061A & 03IS2061E).

The authors would like to thank Prof. Dr. Konrad Ott, Prof. Dr. Heinrich Assel, Prof. Dr. Dr. Mariacarla Gadebusch Bondio and Pia Erdmann M.A for important advice and input. Gratitude is also expressed to Kristin Zielinski M.A. and Sally Werner for support of the compilation of the footnotes.

Can Objections to Individualized Medicine be Justified?

Konrad OTT, Tobias FISCHER

Abstract: The article analyses two strategies of radical criticism towards the field of Individualized Medicine (IM): "Marxist Criticism", which sees IM as nothing more than a construct by the medical and pharmaceutical industries (MPI) to invent new markets, and "Bio-politics according to Foucault", which can be attributed to the fact that every piece of (genetic) knowledge and the state of health might also offer an approach to exercise some power over the individual. By analysing the current route of MPI we find a structure – some might consider it a capitalistic strategy – which rests upon several logical pillars and modules and lets us assume that IM does not lose epistemic plausibility but might benefit the health of the public instead and can therefore be ethically legitimized. In the second part, we show that by bringing up "bio-power" against the concept of IM, Foucault's concept reveals some serious normative deficits. Even more, Foucault's overall philosophy including his "cura sui" and IM do certainly not stand in *opposition* to one another. IM can take a stance in the peculiar dialectics of subjects being individualized by modern medicine on the one hand and exercising and performing self care (*"epimeleia"*) on the other hand.

1 Introduction

In modern societies, every technological innovation seems to bring some critics to the scene: genetic engineering, nanotechnology, nuclear fusion, manned space flight etc. This phenomenon is not simply the expression of an irrational technophobia but can be interpreted as an achievement of a reflexive modernity wherein technological innovations as such do not count as progress any more. Considered empirically, this permanent criticism results in the fact that shaping options of innovation processes are put up for discussion and may become politically negotiable (e.g. nuclear phase-out).[1]

---

[1] Concepts and institutions of technology assessment have also existed since the 1980s. The German Büro für Technikfolgen-Abschätzung (TAB; Office of Technology Assessment at the German Bundestag), for instance, produced an authoritative study on Individualized Medicine (IM), see B. Hüsing, J. Hartig, B. Bührlen, T. Reiß, S. Gaisser (Eds.), *Individualisierte Medizin und Gesundheitssystem*, TAB-Arbeitsbericht 126, Berlin 2008.

173

With this in mind, even radical criticism of Individualized Medicine (IM) is a normal. Critics of IM currently enjoy significant interest in the media and are discussed in the specialized press as well as in feuilletons and science sections: Articles titled "Das große Versprechen" ("The Big Promise") indicate some patterns of this debate and confront optimistic statements of pharmacologists with other voices who consider IM to be a waste of money and warn against false hopes.[2] Said article quotes high-profile critics such as Bärbel Hüsing who describes Individualized Medicine, particularly the field of pharmacogenetics based on biomarkers, as PR tactics. Among others, Regine Kollek suggested that IM can indeed be understood as a health science approach which imposes the duty to care for the preservation or restoration of one's own health.[3] There are legitimate concerns against a tendency toward de-solidarization within the German health insurance system, there might be dangers of a stealthy undermining of the principle of informed consent due to a "gentle pressure to participate", and there might loom a sanctioning of life plans with a certain risk profile in case of non-compliance. Often, such media-debates follow the routines of how to assess risks and benefits and they make the public sphere attentive to IM. We do not address such legitimate concerns in this article. More interesting to us are more radical types of criticism because they are challenging an emerging field as IM in an early stage of development. To face such challenge, we choose two critical approaches which we refer to as "Marxist Criticism" and "Bio-politics according to Foucault" and which this article is concerned with.

"Marxist Criticism" sees IM as hype constructed by the medical and pharmaceutical industries (MPI) to capture or invent new markets with niche preparations without actually benefiting patients.[4] The rationales behind this hype are imperatives of capital accumulation. This approach is strengthened by the realisation that the pharmaceutical industry is in a crisis as there have hardly been any licenses for new blockbuster drugs in the

[2] M. Grill, V. Hackenbroch, "Das große Versprechen", in: *Der Spiegel*, 32/2011, p. 124-128.

[3] U. Hempel, "Personalisierte Medizin I, Keine Heilkunst mehr, sondern rationale molekulare Wissenschaft", in: *Deutsches Ärzteblatt*, 106(42)/2009, p. A-2068, B-1769, C-1733.

[4] W. Bartens, Art. "Jedem seine Pille", in: *Süddeutsche Zeitung* 18.03.2011.

last 20 years and the existing blockbusters are successively superseded by generic drugs[5]. MPI does not even deny this. However, the benefit of IM for patients is clearly emphasized by companies. For instance, Roche announces its new strategy in a promotionally effective way:

"[...] Despite a changing healthcare market and product setbacks this year, Roche is implementing this initiative from a position of strength. In contrast with many of its competitors, Roche's exposure to patent expiries over the next several years is low, and the Group has 14 product franchises, each generating annual sales of more than 1 billion Swiss francs. With its combined strengths in pharmaceuticals and diagnostics and its recognized expertise in molecular biology, Roche is uniquely positioned to advance personalized healthcare solutions, giving patients access to safer, more effective treatment options."[6]

Is IM primarily pushed only as a new capitalisation strategy of the pharmaceutical industry or is it after all a scientific attempt to turn the pharmacological focus increasingly to diagnostic techniques and targeted therapies by using biomarkers and finer possibilities of stratification? What is supposedly wrong with a long-term increase in the provision of medical products and services through innovation and investment? Is it not normal that there will be no investment without sound expectations for returns of investment?

Another field of criticism can be attributed to the fact that every piece of (genetic) knowledge about the state of health of a person might also offer an approach to exercise some power and control in the broadest sense by accessing that knowledge. Scientific knowledge constitutes not only power over nature, as Bacon argued, but it constitutes social power relations as well. If scientists such as the renowned US expert on health innovations, George Poste, speculate almost naively (in the context of the future possibilities of IM) about implanting sensors into the bodies of patients which

---

5   See K. Kaitin, J. A. DiMasi, "Pharmaceutical Innovation in the 21st Century: New Drug Approvals in the First Decade, 2000-2009", in: *Clinical Pharmacology and Therapeutics,* 89(2)/2011, p.183-188; Berger notes: "With more than half of the industry's sales going off-patent within the next three years, 65% of the companies surveyed think the pharmaceutical industry is facing a strategic crisis." (R. Berger, "'Fight or Flight?': Roland Berger Study Intensifies Diversification as One of the Most Prominent Trends in the Pharmaceutical Industry"; http://www.rolandberger.com/media/press/releases/510-press_archive2010_sc_content/Diversification_in_the_pharmaceutical_industry.html).

6   http://www.roche.com/media/media_releases/med-cor-2010-11-17.html.

permanently monitor the state of health and transfer this data via telecommunication to the supervising healthcare system[7], it seems justified to ask what this knowledge – biomarkers, genetic dispositions, health results of all kinds – will be used for within the system. What might full transparency of medical data imply in societal terms? Thomas Lemke has argued against IM within a Foucaultian frame of thought[8]. Overcoming this approach we wish to apply two different concepts to IM, namely the concept of bio-politics and the ethical concept of "cura sui", i.e. the prudent or even wise care for oneself. In the following sections, we wish to analyse these two strategies of criticism in more detail.

In science, criticism must not only be tolerated but should be addressed and disputed. Criticism is never without ethical presuppositions but is based on certain theoretical *frames*. Therefore, a critique can only be appreciated if the respective *frames* have been understood. In philosophy, it is common courtesy to strengthen a critique as much as possible even if one does not share it. We consider the following assumption to be discourse-rationally plausible: A position which has been subject to various critiques but could withstand this criticism successfully can be considered as *confirmed* (in a Popperian sense). *Duplex negatio affirmat:* we adopt this logical principle of double negation ("duplex negatio est affirmatio") for our investigation. Of course, the case of IM is not as easy as in pure (classical) logic, in which the principle holds with respect to single propositions: "the negation of p is true if and only if p is false". The principle must be applied at the far more complex layer of, say, ethical-political epistemology of IM.

2 Criticism of Capitalism and IM

IM is without a doubt part of the scientific context of a medical-pharmaceutical industry (MPI) and therefore also to be seen in the context of the economic imperatives which this sector is subject to. An economic context does not necessarily have to, but might, entail causal impacts on the scientific conception of IM. One perception says that the IM concept primarily originated *within* the realm of scientific medicine and can ultimately

---

[7]   G. Poste, Art. "Richtiges Mittel für die richtige Person", in: *Die Presse* 14.11.2010.

[8]   See T. Lemke (Ed.), *Biopolitik zur Einführung*, Hamburg 2007, Chapters 6-8.

be justified only within this realm; according to this view, the economic context would be *external* to the IM concept. Therefore, economic aspects, which can hardly be denied, only belong to the contingent surroundings of IM, not to the matter itself. Research money from MPI to scientific IM-studies would not change this picture. In this view, research money enables science but does not impair scientific investigation. Another possibility would be that the economic context does not just surround and support IM, but has a verifiable influence on the origin and justification of the conception itself. Most Marxists entertain this hypothesis. For this second perception Marxian critics should be willing to adopt the burden of proof. However, if the corresponding proof could be given, IM concepts would be suspected of being some form of *ideology*. The notion of ideology in the Marxian tradition is conceived as a reflexion of material economic relations in the domains of law, religion, morals, and even science. In this case, the debate would not be about what certain gullible and well-meaning doctors might think and say concerning IM, but about an "objective" explanation of IM based on the economic imperatives of a certain sector of capitalism. The most ambitious Marxist approaches to so-called "Bio-Capitalism"[9] which includes IM, want to furnish this proof.

2.1 If one wants to understand this type of criticism better, some remarks on the theoretical form of Marxism are in order. We take the following hypothesis as a starting point: One can still learn a lot from Marx in an analytical economic respect, but only very little in an ethical respect. Therefore, one can be an analytical-explanatory Marxist and defend at least the social-state varieties of capitalism normatively and politically (thus being a normative anti-communist[10]). Analytical Marxism supposes the moral *need* for legitimisation of all political and economic orders but it does not assume the fundamental illegitimacy of certain e.g. capitalistic orders. An analytical Marxist may concede that, despite all inequalities, the technological dynamism of capitalism will, in the longer run, provide most people at least in the most advanced capitalist societies with the material requisites for a decent and flourishing life. We do not wish to decide such claims but

---

9   See K. S. Rajan, *Biocapital. The Constitution of Postgenomic Life,* Durham/London 2006.

10   A solid overview to contemporary Marxist approaches is given in R. Albritton, R. Jessop, R. Westra (Eds.), *Political Economy and Global Capitalism,* London 2007.

only point at the theoretical possibility that analytic Marxists may support some variants of capitalism.

Marxism has been a peculiar theory from the beginning, which claims on the one hand to be able to analyse, causally explain and partly even predict economic processes (such as crises) in capitalistic societies and which on the other hand features a normative and ethical dimension within which the capitalistic economy is rated and condemned as deeply unjust. In the early writings of Marx and Engels, the ethical dimension is still clearly present (for instance in Marx' so-called Categorical Imperative[11]) but it recedes in the writings of the "mature" and more sober Marx.[12] Later, in the orthodox Marxist/Leninist doctrine of Eastern communist states, the ethical dimension is conceptualized as teleological morality according to which everything that serves the build-up of socialism is "good" and everything that damages or hinders it is "bad"[13]. This teleological ethics allowed actions within Stalinism which are illegitimate, even reprehensible, in a civil-liberal morality (forced labour, show trials, evictions and displacements etc.). The deep moral corruption of communist states is hard to deny. The "blind spot" of Neo-Marxism since the 1970s has been the belief that it had the monopoly on morals and distributive justice, which can unfortunately lead to self-righteousness and even moral arrogance.

2.2 Capitalism is characterized by a) the legal institution of private property on means of production, b) a dynamics of profit orientation, investment activity and accumulation of capital stocks; c) a tendency to model substantial conditions of life (work, accommodation, natural environment, health) according to economic imperatives and d) the market as primary coordination mechanism of economic activity. Prices are signals of relative scarcity which are influenced by increase and restriction of supply and demand. Humans are modelled by mainstream economic science as beings which, on the average, wish to maximize their personal utility in the fields

---

[11] K. Marx, "Zur Kritik der Hegelschen Rechtsphilosophie. Einleitung.", in: Institut für Marxismus-Leninismus beim ZK der SED (Ed.), *Karl Marx Friedrich Engels – Werke*, Volume 1, Berlin 1976, p. 378-391, p. 385.

[12] The relationship of ethics and Marxism is debated in E. Angehrn, G. Lohmann (Eds.), *Ethik und Marx*, Königstein 1986. See esp. the contributions of Wood, Wildt, and Lohmann.

[13] See e.g. the Stalinist writer A. Schischkin, *Die Grundlagen der kommunistischen Moral*, Berlin 1959.

of consumption (pleasure) or production (profit).The concept of rationality is modelled accordingly.

The capitalistic spiral of capital C, investment I, wares W, profit P and capital accumulation C' is endless in principle: $C \rightarrow I \rightarrow W \rightarrow P \rightarrow C' \rightarrow I'$ $\rightarrow W' \rightarrow P' \rightarrow C'' \rightarrow I''$ etc. This spiral is a growth strategy, as the relation is supposed to be $C' > C$, meaning there should be an accumulation of capital over time. This spiral has a globalizing force; it successfully overcomes frontiers in space and cultural barriers. However, there is not "one" capitalism, but there are many variants, i.e. capitalisms, which differ primarily in their sets of regulations and in the transfer systems through which market results are regulated and corrected. Variants of capitalism differ mainly in the quantity and quality of state activity: While in liberalistic variants, this activity is mainly focussed on the protection of private property and the legal execution of economic transactions, with the state thus supposed to be "contracted" and many state services supposed to be "privatized", social state variants correct the market results through diverse taxes, solidarity and transfer systems. While liberal variants see state activities as "distorting" market effects, social-state variants see the same activities as "correcting" market effects for the benefit of the least advanced groups. In the health-care system, this difference between variants is striking, as can be seen in the dispute over the health care reform in the USA. According to the view of the critics of Obama's reform, the German system of health insurance is downright "socialist", while most of us Germans would seem to appreciate it as an achievement of the historically grown social state. Most German citizens, by intuition, defend an egalitarian access to health care services.

2.3 The MPI provides the population of industrialized societies with a broad range of medicines, appliances and services. Individually, these pharmaceuticals and appliances are most impressive. They are innovations which became normality and which are due to today's average patients as a matter of course and thus as background provision. No one doubts that clinics will be well equipped with pharmaceutics and medical technology in the future. Friedrich Dessauer worked out this point very clearly in his "*Philosophie der Technik*"[14]. Medical innovation, paradigmatically the new active ingredient, does not serve a particular person, but is addressed to

---

[14] F. Dessauer (Ed.), *Philosophie der Technik*, Bonn 1927.

many anonymous others. Biomedical research, as "cold" as it may seem at first sight, is carried by an underlying altruistic impulse to be able to provide improved help for future patients. For the patient it is far better if an active ingredient is available than if he is merely nursed lovingly. For most of us, it has become a matter of course that there are X-ray units, low-risk general anaesthetics, antibiotics, ceramic dental fillings, micro-invasive surgery techniques, prostheses etc. and competent and skilled personnel for all these appliances. All these technologies and qualified staff do not simply exist but they are constantly being produced by the medical industry and universities. Leaving persons aside for simplicity, all these medical products keep getting better, but their prices are not true market prices but ultimately politically negotiated prices. These utility or service values have considerably increased the health of the public in capitalistic economies in a long-term perspective. Only a few people would deny that, in effect, the health care of a (German) unemployment benefit claimant today is considerably better than that of an industrial worker, a civil servant or even the Kaiser 150 years ago. Viewed over longer periods of time (and macro-economic theories should have a "historic sense"), a system that combines scientific research, technology development, investment activity, private-sector profit orientation and capital accumulation seems to be superior to all the other known systems in terms of medical performance and, not least due to general wealth, also in terms of inclusion capacity. The right not to be excluded from a health care system can be fulfilled in such system (special cases as illegal immigrants left aside). This assessment gives a certain normative credit to IM as a new option in the system, but does evidently not exclude the possibility *of explaining* IM as a strategy to overcome problems of capital accumulation within such (successful) system.

2.4 In Rajan's writings, the approach to such an explanation is the restricted lifetime of patents and the origin of *generic drugs* as a strategic problem of the pharmaceutical industry. Generic drugs originate because patents on medicines expire. One can now debate whether medicines should be patentable at all. Intuitively, one feels a certain unease since the patenting of medicines complicates the access to them. The following argument speaks for patenting as a moral institution: The ethical legitimacy of the legal institution of the patent is generally not so much the effect of incentive and monetary reward for the inventor as patent-holder, but rather the long-term effect of patenting on the pool of collective knowledge and the better availability of goods. By limiting the patents' lifetime, the amount of collective technological knowledge grows in the longer run. Thus, patents are an institution which links limited monetary rewards (often 20 years) for inventors (today mostly companies) to long-term benefits for the general public.[15] The patent can be seen as a bottleneck of privatization before knowledge pours in the increasing lake of common knowledge. To put it crudely, the blockbusters are both today's money printing machines *and* the cheap generic drugs of the future. Once the patent-protected blockbuster has become a generic drug, it must be substituted by a new profitable product from the point of view of the company concerned. The capital for its development is available. The investment activity is supposed to end in goods yielding high profit rates which are attractive for investors and at the stock exchange, since investors can choose between many alternatives. The capital can either be invested directly in the own company or it can be used to buy and take-over smaller start-up companies which hold attractive patents or are researching promising products.[16] This dynamic field of medical innovations creates opportunities for small-scale entrepreneurship and large companies as well. MPI has to orient its investments in such a way that new products which are superior to the growing stock of generic drugs and can be marketed accordingly are generated. The special thing about the medical industry is that the clientele does not emerge due to the preferences of the customers in free markets but is rather mediated by medicine and the health care system.

2.5 This strategic problem of expiring patents cannot be solved once and for all but it must be processed for the time being. The current route of MPI might consist in a *strategy* that rests upon several pillars and modules: *1) improved response rates of medicines with concurrent reduction of side effects, 2) nosographic extension, 3) extension of threshold values, 4) conception of pre-phases, 5) forward displacement into diagnostics, 6)*

---

[15] Moral problems of the patenting of medicines (e.g. anti-AIDS) appear with reference to Southern countries, for why should people have to die simply because a patent keeps the prices up? A terminally-ill patient cannot wait until the patent has expired.

[16] In this case, it is advantageous if the state sponsors the foundation of companies in close contact with research with tax money, while the industry profitably markets patent-protected medicines and then takes over the successful start-up companies.

adoption of predictive-preventive listings by health insurance companies, 7) additional marketing of products with high symbolic gain of distinction and 8) optimisation of compliance.

Firstly: Up to now, medicines were often produced for mass-markets and widespread diseases when it was clear that they are diseases. The disadvantage of these medicines is that patients respond vastly differently to them, a problem which was until recently solved in a trial-and-error procedure in medical practice. It would be very advantageous for patients if improved information were available in order to reduce unwelcomed side-effects. This stratagem is essentially the most conventional pillar of the strategy as it can link to accepted therapeutic goals with improved means. Even though the means ("virtual copies") may seem utopian, the goals are rather conventional: the "fitting" of medicine for each single patient. Sophisticated diagnostics (e.g. with reference to cancer types) and an extended range of medicines are on the horizon of that goal. Aiming for it is *prima facie* not only ethically allowed, but even to be endorsed. From a utilitarian perspective, it reduces the suffering stemming from side-effects, and from a capability-approach (M. Nussbaum) it improves the capability to stay in good health even under medical treatment.

Secondly the range of what counts as a disease has to be extended. This can be done through the epistemic construction of new diseases and disorders. Recent examples for this strategy of extension are ADHD/Ritalin, depression/Prozac, metabolic syndrome (MS), high blood pressure[17] etc. This strategy of extension meets with the medical research's aim for "good" publications, new external funds for clinical studies[18] and the career imperatives of young scientists. In this stratagem, the concept of disease is complemented by the concept of disorder. Disorders with respect to mental capacities (as memory), digestion, sleep, sex, metabolism etc. become pervasive in recent literature. It is by no means clear epistemologically, whether new disorders are discovered by new scientific findings or whether well-known human phenomena are "seen" as disorders. From a logical point of view,

---

[17] Concerning the relation between high blood pressure and the risk of a stroke, the risk can be increased by the fact that reversible ischemic attacks now count as "true" strokes, which increase the risk of a stroke.

[18] Here, research in population genetics and association and correlation studies play an important role.

any disorder presupposes some range of an orderly state of health. Such range must be determined.

Thirdly, the many threshold values which limit the range of normalcy or "order" have to be stipulated in such a way that the number of persons in need of treatment or monitoring increases. The basic problem is that more and more people are defined into diseases and all sorts of disorders. If, for instance, a cardiogram shows a result which is increased by a few milliseconds compared to the threshold value, medication is advised immediately. The disease of alcoholism can be broadened by defining the criteria more severely; high blood pressure becomes a widespread disease because a low life-long value is stipulated, even though the blood pressure generally increases with age. The stipulation of threshold values and ranges is not simply scientific but rests upon implicit valuations which are often justified by referring to an increase in the *relative* risk – and medical threshold values seem to be covered by the authority of medicine and thus beyond any doubt. The concept of increased relative risk compared to the average of the population serves for the legitimisation of the stipulation of threshold values. Outside the normal range, a person bears a statistically increased risk.[19] This strategy of enlargement of the number of patients and clients by stipulating threshold values does not start with IM, but it could be highly intensified by IM. This is a huge challenge for IM, as these enlargement strategies seem to be highly ambivalent from a medical-ethical point of view. (This strategy implies a close reflection of the attitudes of physicians and on the dialogical counselling relation between physicians and clients. This kind of reflection is beyond the scope of our paper.)

Fourthly, a *pre-phase* can be conceptualized for almost any disease or disorder: pre-osteoporosis, pre-arthrosis, pre-diabetes, pre-dementia, pre-psychosis etc. These pre-phases constitute the different types of the "healthy diseased". People are free of afflictions but on a route which might (or might not) lead to a disease at some point in time. Therefore, IM has to be about gathering pre-clinical results to prevent or delay the onset of diseases. This stratagem is specific to IM. Here, the old medical utopia of preventing disease fuses and blends with new diagnostic strategies.

---

[19] It is often the case that lay people equate a 30% increase in the risk of contracting disease X with a 30% probability of contracting disease X.

Fifthly, the diagnostic sector has to be extended. Medical interventions are moved forward into an area where diagnostics and therapy form a *seamless web.* Among other things, this creates the medical-ethical problem of the valuation of risks of invasive diagnostic procedures. However, this investment strategy is risky as the market for diagnostics carries with it uncertainties on the part of the patients. The entrepreneurial risk of marketing diagnostics thus increases *a fortiori* if the diagnostic technique is invasive. The extension of the diagnostic sector therefore has to be secured by *compliance* strategies (see below).

Sixthly, attempts should be made to get as many IM options as possible into standard health care, but certain extravagant IM products have to be marketed separately as status products. These would then not compete with a standard therapy but with Ayurvedic cures, cruises, a convertible sports car etc. Certain IM products, the consumption of which promises a gain of cultural distinction[20] must not be invoiced via statutory health insurance because they are symbolic status goods which not everyone should be able to afford. Markets for such *high-end IM products* seem to be existent in the group of the affluent elderly people which strive to enjoy many years at high quality of life. Here, IM and wellness are to be combined in luxury products to which one "treats oneself".

Seventhly, the *compliance* of the candidates/patients has to be optimized. Compliance would seem to be a decisive condition for the success of IM. However, this compliance is not very good in today's medicine. Therefore, the strategic problem is to achieve compliance rates for the strategy of the extension of the conventional understanding of disease which are higher than the compliance rates of today's orthodox medicine. These innovations in IM and compliance therefore require a guiding principle or a convincing narrative which causes behavioural changes in the target groups of IM. Since the principle of the voluntariness of all medical interventions cannot simply be suspended in a liberal society (see below), there has to be an appeal to values such as "security", "responsibility" or "the public good". Certainly, compliance can also be increased through economic incentives and especially deterrents.[21] Currently, there are a number of in-

---

[20]   P. Bourdieu, *Die feinen Unterschiede. Kritik der gesellschaftlichen Urteilskraft*, Frankfurt 1987.

[21]   A well-known incentive is the bonus one gets, if one has not seen a doctor for a year.

quiries whether "irresponsible" persons who do not make use of preventive checkups should only be partly reimbursed for the treatment when the disease does break out. These proposals can then be discussed bio-ethically; for instance, is it fair to give such an incentive if the diagnostic technique itself is considered to be risky. We do not further elaborate on these partly medical-ethical, partly health-political questions here.

In summary, it is good for MPI if there are as many clients as possible, i.e. "healthy diseased" and candidates/patients/clients who do not really suffer from new diseases and disorders but show "results" in the pre-clinical range, who have increased values and risks and who are subjected to a continuous diagnostic monitoring as real-potential patients. Thus, the overall strategy of MPI consists of several pillars and many modules which can be combined variably and with a high degree of flexible response. This overall strategy requires a close cooperation with the medical profession and medical research, especially at university hospitals. Its implementation into clinical routines requires a strong *agency network*, i.e. a stable coalition between MPI, scientific medical research and (private) health insurance companies which is based on different but parallel interests and similar epistemic and bioethical convictions. Agency network rely on common interests, convictions, and imaginaries. Therefore, the crucial hypothesis of an analytical-explanatory Marxist could read: IM offers a conceptual epistemic and normative matrix for the implementation of such strategies by a IM agency network.

"Moreover, the *possibility* of Personalized Medicine is *insurance* (for the patient, against future illness), just as the always already existent patient-as-consumer is insurance for the pharmaceutical company. [...]: the patient's risk of future disease is inseparable from the pharmaceutical company's risk of high investment in therapeutic development that must be realized in an eventual commodity. My argument so far has been that a particular discursive-epistemic shift allows a reconfiguration of subject categories away from normality and pathology towards variability and risk, thereby placing *every* individual within a probability calculus as a potential target for therapeutic intervention".[22]

This incentive does not fit in with the IM concept and should be generally forbidden as it contributes to persons seeing a physician too late. It is a so-called perverse incentive.

[22] K. S. Rajan, *Biocapital*, p. 167.

2.6 Assuming that one can concede this analysis as a basic plausibility, would that expose IM as ideology? Believing this would be wrong and misleading for several reasons.

Firstly, the strategy of MPI does not at all exclude the possibility that IM may have a sound epistemic *fundamentum in re*. Too much scientific evidence, most of which cannot simply be declared as "constructs" (on the base of Radical Constructivism) speaks in favour of this. (The idea of a "construct" has an extremely broad extension, therefore little intension, and is mostly used pseudo-critically.) Association studies of IM are expressive in themselves and heuristically productive for a deeper aetiological understanding of diseases. The role of genetic dispositions for diseases is generally hard to contest. From the perspectives of life-world and alternative medicine, it is also plausible to assume that diseases have early stages and pre-phases. The exact time of the onset of a disease is not exactly predictable ("*hora incerta*"), but it can be prognosticated with a high probability that there will be an onset at some point in time. Therefore, the pre-orientation of IM can also be well justified epistemologically. There are too many truths and too many reasonable issues in IM to be able to speak generally of a "capitalist ideology". Furthermore, it cannot be assumed that a complacently corrupt IM would lend itself to such a strategy of capitalist industries. *Secondly*, the existence of a strategy does not exclude the possibility that IM might *in the long run* benefit the majority of the population in a health-care respect. Even if one assumes that, in a system of capitalism, the production of exchange values ("Tauschwert") has a primacy over the production of utility values ("Gebrauchswert"), it could be that a capitalistic economy (perhaps precisely because of the primacy of exchange values!) produces a much broader and higher-quality range of utility values than an alternative economic system which focuses on the production of utility values for more basic needs (and on the boundless discussion about what these basic needs are). It could well be that following the IM strategy in an economically rational way will lead to a renewed significant gain in the health-related quality of life of the average citizen in the not too distant future. *Thirdly*, this analysis does not simply expose the moral questions inherent in IM as an ideology and it does not judge the legitimacy of practising and furthering IM. Therefore, it seems right to assume that through this analysis, IM does not lose epistemic plausibility but instead might benefit the health of the public and can be legitimized ethically.

So what did this analysis achieve? The answer is that it sharpens the *science-ethical* sense for the economic context, for the frames and imaginaries and for the narrative or the discursive dispositive of IM. It is not impermissible for MPI to pursue its economic interests and to design a *persuasive* dispositive in accordance with the advertisement of goods to that end. IM will be advertized nicely by means of PR. It might be contested whether the MPI shall be allowed to attract customers through advertisement, as any other industry does. But such permission, if given to MPI, does not hold for medicine. In the case of medicine, fundamentally different rules apply due to its Hippocratic tradition, its basal form of ethics and the widely acknowledged principles[23]. Through the economic imperatives and through advertising strategies of MPI, IM gains new ethical requirements. IM comes at the price of deeper epistemological and ethical questioning. Ironically, an analytical Marxian approach to IM must plead for epistemology and ethics and therefore concede that ethics can be more than mere ideology.

3 Foucault, "bio-power" and "cura sui"

A critique prevalent among intellectuals concerning the modern health care system draws on the work of Michel Foucault and especially on his concept of "bio-power"[24]. "Bio-power is usually understood as the controlling, disciplining, normalising effects of (semi)governmental institutions and organisations (hospitals, prisons, public health departments etc.) to the bodily-mediated behaviour patterns of people that are *individualized* by this access (records, testimonials, stored data etc.). Foucault's concept of individualization means the *transparency* of single persons by storage of personal data in different media. Ironically, Foucaultians can accept the term "IM" according to their terminology. This is clearly not the notion of individuality, as given by W. v. Humboldt and the Romantic tradition. In this

---

[23]   See T. L. Beauchamp, J. F. Childress, *Principles of Biomedical Ethics*, [6]Oxford 2009.

[24]   See e.g. T. Lemke, *Biopolitik* and T. Lemke, *Gouvernementalität und Biopolitik*, Wiesbaden 2008.

tradition, individuality must be performed within the course of life, while transparency of data is opened up to the eyes of observers. We follow Foucault's definition but are not happy with it.

According to Foucault, bio-power and related bio-politics do not suppress personhood but constitute individual personhood by using a set of documentation techniques. Analyses of bio-power which also consider IM are mostly carried out with a critical, exposing and politically judgemental undertone. In the following paragraphs, this strategy of criticism shall be criticized immanently and ultimately brushed against the grain. Foucault's late ethical work shall be made productive for IM by considering the problem of bio-power with respect to individual care for oneself ("cura sui"). We want to show, firstly, that the concept of bio-power has serious normative deficits and, secondly, that IM can be considered from a *cura sui* perspective with profits for the ethical dimension of IM. Finally, we want to show that the ethics of Foucault's late work and IM are in a complementary relation with one another. In a nutshell: Overcoming rhetoric, IM does not need to fear Foucault's overall philosophy.

In Foucault's work,[25] three epistemological interests are distinguished, which can be roughly assigned to certain work phases: The first interest is oriented in an epistemological-historical way. Foucault deals with scientific classification systems e.g. in psychiatry[26] or with epistemic figurations in the humanities[27]. The value of these publications for the history of science is not discussed here. The second interest concerns connections between the generation of knowledge and the function of organisations such as hospitals and prisons[28]. The third interest is divided in itself: It is of a

---

[25] We rely on: A. Honneth, M. Saar (Ed.), *Michel Foucault. Zwischenbilanz einer Rezeption,* Frankfurt 2003. See especially the contributions of Fraser, Lemke, Menke, and Hesse. Important comments on Foucault's philosophy are to be found in J. Habermas, *Der Philosophische Diskurs der Moderne*, Frankfurt a. M. 1984; A. Honneth, *Kritik der Macht,* Frankfurt a. M. 1985; G. Deleuze (Ed.), *Foucault*, Frankfurt a. M. 1987 M. Foucault, "Technologien des Selbst", in: M. Foucault, R. Martin, L. H. Martin, W. E. Paden, K. S.Rothwell, H. Gutman, P. H. Hutton (Eds.), *Technologien des Selbst*, Frankfurt 1993; H.-H. Kögler, *Die Macht des Dialogs,* Stuttgart 1992, part II.

[26] M. Foucault, *Wahnsinn und Gesellschaft. Eine Geschichte des Wahns im Zeitalter der Vernunft,* [10]Frankfurt a. M. 1993.

[27] M. Foucault, *Die Ordnung der Dinge. Eine Archäologie der Humanwissenschaften*, Frankfurt a. M. 2003.

[28] M. Foucault, *Die Geburt der Klinik. Eine Archäologie des ärztlichen Blicks*, Frank-

political and an ethical nature. In his late work, Foucault turns towards the "*cura sui*" conception of antiquity (Greek: "epimeleia") and thus implicitly towards eudaimonistic ethics, i.e. the question of the good and flourishing human life. Foucault takes this turn as philosopher, not as historian. Concerning the politically relevant basic terms of Foucault, he distinguishes between the concepts of power, government and authority. Another part is played by the so-called techniques of the self, by which human beings create themselves as ethical persons.[29] This is where the eudaimonistic concept of "self-concern" comes into play. We shall first of all deal with Foucault's theory of power.

3.1 Foucault: "In my analysis of power, there are three levels: strategic relations, government techniques and authority conditions"[30]. This quote is to be interpreted as follows: On the one hand, there is power in a broad sense, with the broad idea of power comprising all three levels. On the other hand, the idea of power, or rather, of *power relations* in a stricter sense refers to strategic interactions in which "one subject tries to direct the behaviour of another"[31]. According to Lemke[32], power relations are strategic games between at least two actors who try to influence each other[33]. Therefore, power is neither a substance nor a subject; hence, saying that "the" bio-power is doing something is at best to be understood as abbreviating speech; otherwise, it is misleading. Power must not be reified as an object since it is performed, exercized, and executed by actors within interactions.[34] Rather, persons are striving to influence one another effectively by strategic means under certain circumstances and in certain respects. There is no power without the exercise of power.

---

furt a. M. 1976; M. Foucault, *Überwachen und Strafen. Die Geburt des Gefängnisses*, [13]Frankfurt a. M. 1993.

29 M. Foucault, "Technologien des Selbst", in: L. H. Martin, H. Gutman u. P. H. Hutton (Eds.), *Technologien des Selbst*, Frankfurt 1993, p. 24-62.

30 M. Foucault, "Freiheit und Selbstsorge", in: H. Becker (Ed.), *Michel Foucault: Freiheit und Selbstsorge*, Frankfurt a. M. 1985, p. 27.

31 M. Foucault, "Freiheit und Selbstsorge", p. 27.

32 T. Lemke, *Gouvernementalität und Biopolitik*, p. 41.

33 See also: G. Deleuze, *Foucault*, p. 99-130; H.-H. Kögler, *Die Macht des Dialogs*, p. 198-208.

34 Poor pupils of Foucault can be recognized by the fact that they constantly speak of "the" bio-power as if it were a separate subject.

Power is always implied if person A wants to "direct" (control, manipulate, restrict, motivate etc.) person B's behaviour (or if both of them want to "direct" person C's behaviour etc.). The idea of action which is used by Foucault is clearly the concept of strategic action which presupposes freedom and intelligence on both sides of the interactive process[35]. In this concept of action, the terms of intentionality, will and purpose are postulated. It cannot be ruled out that A wants to direct B's behaviour in B's best interest, i.e. that A is selfless ("altruistic") according to his self-conception. Strategic action in another's best interest is conceptually possible. Altruistic action is strategic, for instance, if B is persuaded into an action which he would not carry out voluntarily but which ultimately benefits him. This form of altruistic-strategic action is central to educational practice and a paternalistic medical ethics – and worth considering with respect to IM. If a doctor advises a patient to start a therapy or a diet, this is, to Foucault, a bio-power relation *ex definitione*; likewise, if the school physician advises the children to brush their teeth regularly, if physicians recommend compliance etc.

Power relations are thus defined as strategic interactions in institutional contexts. The categories of power are therefore regulations of random actions and random actors[36]. This implies that power relations are ubiquitous, reciprocal, flexible, unstable, reversible etc. and that there are turn-arounds, twists, directional changes and resistances[37]. Furthermore, there are always options for each party to resist the exercise of power, to avoid it, to redirect or circumvent it: A may believe to have B firmly "in the palm of his hand", while he is already dominated by B without realising it. Power "tricks" and can be "tricked" which is why Foucault compared power struggles to judo. Resistance is to be understood rather in a physical or psychological than in a normative or political way; A meets with resistance in B and has to cope with said resistance. The fact that this idea of resistance became politically "charged" does not change anything about the fact that in Foucault's work, it first figured in the diagrams of forces who want to exert power on one another: Power is a relation of strength.[38]

---

[35] M. Foucault, "Freiheit und Selbstsorge", p. 27.
[36] G. Deleuze, *Foucault*, p. 101.
[37] G. Deleuze, *Foucault*, p. 103.

Ceteris paribus, the ideas of power and resistance are completely value-free. Foucault's idea of power relations is therefore a general concept of interaction which is only subject to the criterion of success of an action and otherwise normatively undefined or "empty". A problem lies in the fact that Foucault's idea of power does not offer any possibilities to distinguish between a well-meant, honest piece of advice and the application of subtle force. Hence, the exercise of power can be distinguished according to degrees of subtlety (and medical advice would be more subtle than compulsory admission to a psychiatric ward), but it cannot be normatively criticized; maybe sophisticated, subtle pressure is more devious than an open, "unvarnished" threat.[39] However this may be, nobody can be morally accused or blamed just by referring to the concept of power. It has been argued by many scholars that Foucault's philosophy is full of critical rhetoric but is devoid of any normative yardsticks that might substantiate all the moral and political suggestions in Foucault's writings. This lack of yardsticks would not matter if one reads Foucault as a historian only.

Foucault is also interested in the question of how scientific knowledge can be applied in strategic interactions, i.e. how power relations make recourse to such knowledge. That this is happening is beyond doubt. If A wants to motivate B to behave in a certain way, A can for instance refer to the authority of science or to the results of evidence-based studies, unmistakeable X-ray images, established medical treatments, the scientific literature in peer-reviewed journals etc. The authority of science, to which an orientation towards truth has to be ascribed in a transcendental-pragmatic way[40], can be used within the functional circle of strategic power. Doubting that, would be naïve. Therefore, one can meaningfully ask which power effects *may* result from bio-banking, clinical routines, genetic diagnoses, stratifications etc.[41]. The many questions of how to cope with such effects

---

[38] M. Foucault, *Dispositive der Macht. Über Sexualität, Wissen und Wahrheit*, Berlin 1978, p. 70.

[39] Furthermore, it is no longer possible to speak of a humanisation of the exercise of power: the modern panoptic prison is a different form of governmental exercise of power or authority than a public execution, but Foucault does not give universal principles which allow a judgement about the question whether life-long imprisonment is "more humane" than public quartering.

[40] K. Ott, *Ipso Facto. Zur ethischen Begründung normativer Implikate wissenschaftlicher Praxis*, Frankfurt a. M. 1997.

in a responsible manner will be the task of IM-bioethics and law.

As a science historian, one can of course prove that the genesis of scientific knowledge[42], e.g. in psychiatry, was interwoven in multiple ways with power relations and also with authority relations. Similarly, it can be shown that vegetation research flourished in the context of the construction of the motorways in the German Reich, that ethnology and colonialism entered into close connections, that genetics was politicized eugenically and that regional planning was politicized imperialistically.[43] However, these political contexts into which science moved either voluntarily or was harnessed *nolens volens,* do not say everything about the contents of the contextually generated knowledge. Foucault realises that, as well: "This fact does not at all touch on the scientific validity or the therapeutic truth of psychiatry. It does not guarantee it, but does not take it back, either."[44]

Deleuze tried to determine the relation between power and scientific knowledge in Foucault's work in a relational-logical way: "Between power and knowledge, there is a fundamental difference, heterogeneity; but also mutual presupposing and mutual co-opting; and finally the primacy of the one over the other"[45]. This succession of relational-logical words is at best awkward, at worst confused, but in any case analytically deficient. Foucault himself put it thus: "Between techniques of knowledge and strategies of power, there is no exteriority, even if they have specific roles and are linked together on the basis of their difference."[46] What Foucault wants to claim is the presence of an *internal* relation between power and knowledge. This hypothesis is plausible and Foucault's historical investigations can be interpreted as empirical studies to confirm this hypothesis. Internal relations are those in which a description or narrative of A would be significantly incomplete without the description of B. Presupposing an internal relation, verbs such as "co-opt" and "join together" can be introduced to specify this internal relation. This should also be possible for IM and deserves examination. But it seems fair to say that Foucault never became philosophically

[41]   See T. Lemke, *Gouvernementalität.*
[42]   K. R. Popper: *"context of discovery"*
[43]   In this respect, us Germans are particularly marked.
[44]   M. Foucault, "Freiheit und Selbstsorge", p. 23.
[45]   G- Deleuze, *Foucault*, p. 103.
[46]   M. Foucault, *The History of Sexuality. An Introduction*, Volume 1, NY 1990, p. 98.

clear about the many kinds and subtypes of intrinsic relations. Foucault's logic does not go very deep.

Terminologically, Foucault distinguishes between power relations and authority relations. The term of authority refers to permanent institutionalized and genuinely political forms of the exercise of power. In its mainstream, political philosophy assumes that political authority as a special form of power exercise highly requires legitimisation. Thus, it asks for the conditions of legitimacy of political authorities and ultimately always finds the answer in the idea of democracy (cf. for instance John Rawls and Jürgen Habermas). However, Foucault does not want to pose the question of the *conditions of legitimacy* of political authority within this liberal mainstream of political philosophy. He does not want to consider authority within normative, political and legal categories but obviously, following Nietzsche, with reference to "life". To this end, he coins and uses the concept of bio-power. Within this concept, the terminological difference between power and authority should be kept but has been conflated often.

According to Foucault, bio-politics is a field in which state's authorities address topics as health, fertility, sports, diets, migration, and morbidity of whole populations and single persons. Bio-politics can refer to single individuals and can exercise power on them, but it can also refer to populations in order regulate them[47]. Bio-politics originates in the age of enlightenment, has been continued in the Fordist period of capitalism[48] but now takes a new shape. According to Foucault, modern bio-power, understood as a strategy of the exercise of power in the field of bio-politics, does no longer employ brutal, but rather gentle means; it no longer threatens with internment, but advertises the advantages and the value of security. It does not refer to metaphysical authorities but to scientific knowledge. For decades, it has been pointedly liberal and respects the condition of informed consent. Modern bio-power always has a smile on its face. It encourages bio-ethical discourses and approves of discursive-participative arrangements, patient groups, ethical committees etc. By now, sociologists, psychologists, ethicists, theologians etc. are almost regularly included in research programs. In recent times, individuals do not turn into passive recipients of medical

---

[47] T. Lemke, "Andere Affirmationen", p. 273.
[48] See N. Fraser, "Von der Disziplin zur Flexibilisierung?".

directives, but active, responsible and even opinionated players in the medical power relations. Thus, patients are conceded quite a lot of power in current IM contexts. Perhaps, IM could give more power to client stakeholder groups whose members claim to be experts for their disease or disorder. IM can give voice to the directly concerned.

A strategy of criticism which presents all this as nothing more than wilful deception by cynical bio-political elites would seem highly implausible. Considered systematically, it would be an error theory as it would have to assert that the involved parties fundamentally deceive themselves concerning the things they do and say: That they only believe that they participate in the responsible shaping of medical innovations and are "in reality" character masks of "the" bio-power. However, this error theory assumes a large burden of proof and has to insinuate that the actors fundamentally deceive themselves about what they do. Furthermore, in such reasoning "the" bio-power is personified or reified, which terminologically does not fit Foucault's meaning. Therefore, a strategy of criticism based on Foucault is faced with the alternative of either practising some form of micrology of power relations in the IM sector in a sociological way or developing a normatively content-full critique of IM. Since the concept of bio-power is normatively empty, one can conceive a somewhat critical perspective on IM out of Foucault's writing but not derive bioethical yardsticks that may substantiate and warrant judgments on IM-practices. This perspective should be compatible with the persons that perform IM.

Foucault acknowledged[49] that modern medicine and bio-politics in a broad sense have advantages for humans because it pushes back the constant threat of death which was typical for pre-modern societies. The scourge of humanity, apart from war, is mostly hunger and epidemics. In the 20th century, wars were waged with ever increasing numbers of human casualties but this circumstance does not *per se* speak against the fight against hunger and disease by modern bio-politics. Bio-politics promises longevity due to vaccinations, surgery and anaesthetic techniques, antibiotics, social hygiene, canalisation of potable water, food control, designation of open spaces and recreational areas, and much more.[50] Yes, there has been a broad

---

[49] See M. Foucault, *The History of Sexuality*.

[50] Foucault was not interested in environmental and nature conservation, but the social-hygiene movement can be interpreted as a variant of bio-politics; nudist movement,

stream of political governance schemes in the last three centuries which addressed health conditions, sanitation, diets, sex and proliferation, working conditions, sportive activities, recreation and the like of populations. Why not dub this broad field "bio-politics"? But why oppose modern bio-politics in general?

According to Foucault's premises, bio-politics can never be devoid of power but therefore, it does not need to want to be powerless as long as it can presume and prove to serve a human life which is as long and as healthy as possible. Due to modern bio-politics, Europe passes through the demographic transition from high birth and death rates (18th century) via high birth and decreasing death rates (19th century) towards low birth and death rates (20th century). The probability of dying early (for instance as a woman in childbirth or as a child from diphtheria) has decreased sharply. "[D]eath was ceasing to torment life so directly. [...]: a relative control over life averted some of the imminent risks of death."[51] An early, "untimely" death occurs less frequently. By now, it is almost normal that a person should reach 80 years of age. A death at the age of 70 seems premature.

Through and in the wake of bio-politics, we are learning more about diseases and health than ever before. Through social hygiene and improved food supply as well as gradual reduction of the risks of accidents, average life expectancy increases. At the beginning of the 21st century, IM continues from there with the prospect of an increase in the health-related quality of life combined with a further increase in life expectancy. Increasing life expectancy and the number of "good" years means to benefit the life of humans. Bio-power can thus claim responsibility for being a life-supporting beneficial force. The fact that this requires certain power techniques can hardly be criticized from a Foucaultian perspective since the power does not suppress, but instead produces, supports, and strengthens. Thus, it might enhance vitality and health.

Foucault has to take up certain connotations in the concept of life in order to be able to criticise normalising and disciplining tendencies of bio-

---

sports movement, the German youth hostel and "Wandervogel" movements, life reform, sexual education etc. also belong to "bio-politics" in a broad sense.

[51] See M. Foucault, *The History of Sexuality*, p. 142. Foucault fell prey to a new epidemic. By now, medical progress has made it possible to treat HIV as a serious infection which one does not have to die from as long as one has access to the medicines.

politics. Finally, on the normative level, he counter-poses Nietzschean vitalism to the normalising bio-politics. "[L]ife as a political object was in a sense taken at face value and turned back against the system that was bent on controlling it."[52] In the discursive dispositive of bio-politics, all parties refer to "life": The bio-political party (in an Apollonian way) refers to its capabilities for prolonging and maintaining an average life in good health for a long time, while Nietzschean vitalism (in a Dionysian way) celebrates the "sparkling" life with all its ecstasies and escapades, its resistance and renitence, its pleasures and tempers. This repeats Nietzsche's anarchic aversion to taming of any sort. However, on a bioethical and bio-political level, this aversion is a weak discursive bastion against the promises which modern and post-modern bio-medicine has to offer. Insofar, Foucault's political critique of bio-politics ends with the realisation that these powers can likewise and not without reason refer to life. In the large discursive dispositive, the Nietzschean rebels take the position of outsiders.[53] And why should one rule out that a life which is long and healthy should be lived very intensively? It might also be the case that IM reduces the risks of an intensively lived life, that in an upcoming IM paradigm, an intensively enjoyed life does not mean that the candle of life burns at both ends.

Ultimately, a normative critique of IM is not possible from a Foucaultian perspective of power. This is most evident in the attempt to articulate it.[54] Lemke offers an analogy between traditional medicine and the police's protection against threats on the one hand and IM and the undercover practice of the secret service on the other hand. According to Lemke, IM operates in a realm of shadows. As Lemke says, in the paradigm of prevention, there are only shadows: the subject as a shadow of itself, a bundle of susceptibility in a realm of shadows.[55] This is nothing but associative rhetoric and it says more about the critic than about the item being criticized. Lemke himself seems to be aware of the ambivalences of IM, but he

---

[52] See M. Foucault, *The History of Sexuality*, p. 144.
[53] Approaches which want to promote the happiness or the good life of all human beings be they utilitarian or Aristotelian, do not have to oppose bio-politics. Kantians and contractualists can come to terms with modern bio-politics and IM as long as certain principles are maintained.
[54] T. Lemke, *Gouvernementalität*, p. 171.
[55] T. Lemke, *Gouvernementalität*, p. 171.

writes that due to the interest in differences and variations, rigid regulations of normality might lose importance especially in the IM context. Not every deviation, every result, every disposition would have to be regarded as being pathological. And Lemke cannot fail to see the fact that persons no longer want to passively subject themselves to IM but claim a say in initiatives. Thus, in Lemke's publication, there remains not much more than the prosaic assertion that the term of self-determination had contracted, and the concern against a genetic reductionism which is not entailed in IM necessarily.

3.2 In view of the normative deficits, Foucault's turn towards the conception of "*cura sui*" is less surprising than it seems. The path into eudaimonistic ethics remains open even if the normative strategy of criticism can no longer free itself from its deficits and aporiae. Foucault took his final turn as an ethicist, not as an historian. The care for oneself, which precedes self-awareness, was understood as *epimeleia* in antiquity. To Foucault, this is an attitude which was schematized in the Hellenistic period after the model of medicine and which can be determined as constant healthwise care.[56] The attitude of *epimeleia* implies that one becomes one's own physician[57]. This presupposes the perception of the healing arts as *techne* and also as *eupraxia*. Practicing the role of the good doctor to oneself, i.e. becoming one's own therapist, requires certain techniques such as writing, *askesis*, temporary withdrawal from social life, but also dream interpretation and the cleansing of the conscience. In *epimeleia,* dietetics, hygiene and sexual education (not sexual "morals") are incorporated. In this sense, *epimeleia* can be described as "holistic". It is closer to today's human-ecological and "alternative" medical approaches than to orthodox medicine. *Epimeleia* must be exercized. Therefore, if there is always bio-politics being exercized on individual subjects, subjectivity emerges by *epimeleia* being exercized by the subjects themselves throughout their lives[58].

To Foucault, the opposite of *epimeleia* is, in Latin wording, *stultitia*, i.e. folly. A fool is someone whose existence disperses in time, who does

---

[56] M. Foucault, "Technologien des Selbst", p. 41.

[57] M. Foucault, "Technologien des Selbst", p. 41.

[58] C. Menke, "Zweierlei Übung. Zum Verhältnis sozialer Disziplinierung und ästhetischer Existenz", in: A. Honneth, M. Saar (Eds.), *Michel Foucault. Zwischenbilanz einer Rezeption*, Frankfurt a. M. 2003, p. 283-299.

not care for anything, not even himself, and whose will is changeable and erratic. However, in Stoics, *epimeleia* always has the purpose of preparation for evils such as strokes of fate, diseases and, ultimately, death. Insofar, it contributes to a healthy life *and* to the preparation for diseases which shall be borne with indifference ("*ataraxia*"). The ideal of Stoics is the emotional calmness in the face of mundane incidents. (Modern medicine would probably rather welcome stoic virtues in patients).

Epimeleia, as exercise, is self-care, which implies self-devotion. It is an attitude of attention and devotion towards oneself and others which is epitomized by certain practices. These are the so-called *Practices of Self*. These practices promote the attentive devotion to oneself without objectifying oneself. Foucault believes to find in *epimeleia* a form of care for oneself which is not committed to a Cartesian body-mind-dualism or a conception of self-disciplining. One can't exercise *epimeleia* out of the attitude of obedience to another person. In performing *epimeleia*, the concept of bio-power becomes pointless. By such self-caring exercise, one might come to *trust* one's own vital body. This trusting is something other than permanent self-monitoring using apparatuses and devices. In the attitude of *epimeleia*, one does not monitor oneself in one's bodily functions but treats oneself in one's vital corporeality in a friendly and trusting way. The body appears trust-worthy in its vital disposition to maintain and regain health.

3.3 What, then, is the relation between *epimeleia* and IM? To Lemke[59] IM is a regime of truth, a set of power strategies and a new context for practices of self. However, it is terminologically misguided to draw on the idea of power with reference to self-care. Self-care is no power relation in the sense defined by Foucault. It would be conceptually absurd and misleading to initially divide the person (for instance into the "good core" and the "weaker self") in order to then let that divided personality stage internal power games with "itself". This is neither the ancient sense of *epimeleia* nor its understanding in Foucault's work.

However, Lemke comes upon an important point, as IM could mislead into conceptualising *epimeleia* as a permanent form of self-monitoring which must be continually improved by technological means. There are indeed tendencies towards this, one example being the idea of the chip which

---

[59] See T. Lemke, *Biopolitik*, p. 130.

is implanted under the skin and constantly transmits certain bodily results to a database.

However, *epimeleia*, understood as an attitude and practical exercise, is not self-monitoring, but rather awareness and trust in oneself.[60] We understand *epimeleia* or self-care as the epitome of an ensemble of related therapeutic and transformative practises of attentive self-devotion. Self-care is performative self-therapeutics. Every individual has this ensemble to choose from and it is unproblematic if she chooses the practices which she intuitively thinks (or "feels") will suit her. Practises of self are exercized voluntarily. IM could approve of and promote practices of self which are not to reduced to the fastidious "scanning" of the body for signs of disease: The concentration in archery, the eroticism of Tango, the meditation techniques of yoga, the healthful relaxation while listening to music, the writing of a diary, the cleansing of the skin in a steam bath, contacts with nature, picnics with friends, the preparation of good food, therapeutic fasting, restful holidays etc. are therapeutic practices in a (very) broad sense[61] which are obviously not medicinal in a narrow sense but which could be concretized (*"concrescere"*) by the possible combination of human ecology, "alternative" medicine and IM.

4 Outlook

IM can emerge from these two strategies of criticism both strengthened *and* changed. These and further critiques compel IM to reflect about its own understanding of itself, which is not simply fixed, but needs to be developed further. As we feel to have shown, it would be foolish to dread this critique or to discredit it polemically. To draw on Hegel, a lot can be learned about a subject if one has learned to face its negativity (commercial strategies, bio-politics) patiently. Ultimately, this inconvenient compulsion benefits IM. With respect to MPI, IM should not fell prey to commercial interests. Sober scepticism against rosy promises seems appropriate. IM

---

[60] The "self" in this case is no independent substance ("Self") but only has the grammatical purpose of the reference to the respective own existence.

[61] We leave open the question whether "good" sex should be considered to be a therapeutic practice.

should not give Marxists compelling reasons to argue in favour of IM as capitalistic ideology.

With respect to Foucault's philosophy, IM and *epimeleia* could be practized complementarily: Preventive IM, which aims for well-tolerated and suitable therapies in a strict sense, and a careful and attentive self-devotion in self-therapeutic practices in a broad sense do certainly not stand in *opposition* to one another and do thus not preclude one another logically, terminologically or in life praxis. IM has to take a stance in the peculiar dialectics of subjects being individualized and disciplined by modern medicine on the one hand, exercising and performing *epimeleia* on the other hand. To take a conceptual stance is logically independent from the empirical matter that only few people are exercising *epimeleia*. An ethical culture of IM would not only tolerate and respect *epimeleia*, but would recommend and support it as both attitude and exercise. By doing so, it restricts a scientific-technological attitude from within. Dialectical relations can be specified to new and, perhaps, unusual combinations of IM and *epimeleia*. Such combinations are to be exercized in an experiential and experimental manner. We feel some initial sympathies with this perspective, but restrict ourselves to such outlook which must be substantiated within a comprehensive philosophy of IM.

Acknowledgements

This work is part of the research project Greifswald Approach to Individualized Medicine (GANI_MED). The GANI_MED consortium is funded by the Federal Ministry of Education and Research and the Ministry of Cultural Affairs of the Federal State of Mecklenburg-Western Pomerania (support codes: 03IS2061A & 03IS2061E).

The authors are grateful to Margarita Berg for the translation of the article.

Person at Genetic Risk? Ethical and Social Challenges in Individualized Medicine

Matthias BRAUN, Jens RIED

Abstract: The discussions on the so-called Individualized Medicine, its chances, possibilities and visions shape the present debates on the future of medicine and health care. Apart from fundamentally questioning what the actual subject of such an *individualized* medicine is, there are again and again ethical concerns and queries, that are invoked against the so-called Individualized Medicine. In this article, these critical questions, as well as the challenges and chances of the so-called Individualized Medicine will be illuminated from an ethical perspective. At that, it has to be stated that the so-called Individualized Medicine is primarily about accompanying the current developments with an ethical assessment; however, there are presently no ethical arguments that speak against further research in this field per se. The questions in the field of the so-called individualized medicine can rather be integrated into the classical questioning of medical ethics such as public health research.

1 Introduction

'Individualized', 'personalized' or 'customized': The choice of paraphrases and descriptions for the (allegedly) new approach in medicine oscillates and evokes hopeful expectations as well as many times a sceptical look. In spite of on-going attempts of definitions in the most various disciplines and first successes, especially in oncology, there has been no suggestion able to gain broad acceptance so far.[1] Thus it often remains unclear what exactly is meant by the so-called Individualized Medicine.[2] On the background of

---

[1] R. Damm, "Personalisierte Medizin und Patientenrechte – Medizinische Optionen und medizinrechtliche Bewertung", in: *Medizinrecht*, 29/2011, p. 7-17.

[2] See B. Hüsing, J. Hartig, B. Bührlen, T. Reiß, S. Gaisser (Eds.), *Individualisierte Medizin und Gesundheitssystem*, TAB-Arbeitsbericht 126, Berlin 2008, p. 7: Here, Individualized Medicine is provisionally defined in a functional way as "eine mögliche künftige Gesundheitsversorgung [...], die aus dem synergistischen Zusammenwirken der drei Treiber 'Medizinischer und gesellschaftlicher Bedarf', 'Wissenschaftlich-technische Entwicklungen in den Lebenswissenschaften' und 'Patientenorientierung' entstehen könnte".

such a lack of interpretative clarity and presently highly diverging scenarios regarding the question which consequences the approach of the so-called Individualized Medicine will have for the individual patient, the relationship between patients and their doctors, as well as the progression of the health care system as a whole, ethics are challenged to gauge risks as well as chances of this development. In the following, such an assessment will be outlined according to seven ethical challenges in discourse, looking at the so-called individualized medicine in the sense of a "vision assessment"[3] of new technologies and biomedical trends.

2 Individualized Medicine – Trapped by Language Policy?

If the so-called Individualized Medicine wants to do more than just stating a lack of patient orientation in the daily routine in hospitals, it has to be clarified to what individualization or personalization it refers. This is especially valid if the reference to the individual is built upon biomarker-differentiations[4] and thus primarily on scientifically refined medicine, but not on the so-called talking medicine, which is strongly demanded. Occupying the term 'personality' for scientific measures of differentiation is at least prone to misunderstanding. Since personality develops only in social interaction according to a broad stream of theological, philosophical and psychological traditions,[5] personality and communication with the other are mutually conditioned. Accordingly, the term 'personalized medicine'

---

[3] See J.Grin, A. Grunwald (Eds.), *Vision Assessment: Shaping Technology in 21st Century Society: Towards a Repertoire for Technology Assessment*, Berlin/NY 2000.

[4] See B. Hüsing, J. Hartig, B. Bührlen, T. Reiß, S. Gaisser (Eds.), *Individualisierte Medizin und Gesundheitssystem*, TAB-Arbeitsbericht 126, Berlin 2008, p. 8: "Im Kontext der individualisierten Medizin wird insbesonders an die Genom- und Postgenomforschung, die molekulare medizinische Forschung und die zellbiologische Forschung die Erwartung gerichtet, eine Wissens- und Technologiebasis bereitzustellen, von der aus verbesserte Diagnose-, Therapie- und Präventionsmöglichkeiten entwickelt werden können".

[5] In the English-speaking tradition the notion of 'person' is connoted very differently, here the main focus lies on conscience and possession. Though these connotations become more and more important, the mentioned connotations oriented at dialogue remain plausible but they have to have become a stronger part of the public consciousness again; see J. Heinrichs, K. Stock, Art. "Person", in: TRE, Vol. 26, Berlin/Boston 1996, p. 220-231.

has to be understood as especially infelicitously chosen, if it does not imply a medicine oriented towards dialogue, but a medicine relying on refined biomedical processes.

Dispensing with the epithet 'personalized' and alternatively reverting to terms like 'customized' or 'individualized' evokes the problem that at present we cannot speak of a truly *individualized* medicine in the sense of an exactly fitting medicine for each and every patient regarding biomedical and economical facts.[6] On a biomedical level, the sequencing and mapping of the human genome has opened up the access to molecular medicine; but it has become obvious how extremely complex the cross-linking within the genome, between the genomes, the intra-organismic surroundings and the extra-organismic environment is. Achieving an exactly fitting individualization of diagnostics and therapy in this interaction is extremely difficult, extremely time-consuming and extremely expensive. Thus, not only the respective parts of the individual genome would have to be sequenced, which is – despite dropping costs – still too expensive,[7] but also other lifestyle factors would constantly have to be checked and observed in order to note the differences over the pass of time. Establishing such an approach in the context of broad public health care is economically hardly neither imaginable nor presentable, so that the promise of a true individualization is too boastful and can only disappoint, regarding the current point of research.

If willed to do without the respective terms, without giving up on the idea of an exactly fitting medicine with better therapeutic effect and fewer side effects, it is advisable to prefer more realistic alternatives that are more modest on the level of language, such as 'stratified' or 'stratifying' medicine.[8] Furthermore, many results of trust research support such a procedure that is not that prone to betrapped by language policy. Thus, generating public trust in a new, complex technological development is most

---

[6] See B. Hüsing et al., *Individualisierte Medizin und Gesundheitssystem*; M. Gadebusch Bondio, S. Michl, "Die neue Medizin und ihre Versprechen", in: *Deutsches Ärzteblatt*, 107(21)/2010, A-1062, B-934, C-922.

[7] What remains to be investigated is the extent to which the visions of synthetic biology, the development of the so-called Individualized Medicine can be considerably promoted and will be realizable. See E. D. Green, S. M. Guyer, "Charting a Course for Genomic Medicine from Base Pairs to Bedside", in: *Nature*, 470/2011, p. 204–213.

[8] N. Siegmund-Schultze, "Personalisierte Medizin in der Onkologie: Fortschritt oder falsches Versprechen?", in: *Deutsches Ärzteblatt*, 108(37)/2011, p. A-1904.

sustainable if the expectations launched are realistic.[9] When communicating such scientific results and projects, the complexity of the matter has to be taken into account and despite the possibly high financial and ideal aid of resources the risk of possible failure has to be mentioned. If this vision (as a realistic one) shows better prospects compared to the current situation, this process can be of social value, in spite of the possibly stony path thereto.[10] Since the term 'Individualized Medicine' is preferred in the discourse so far and this article deals with the present ethical challenges of exactly this phenomenon, the presented irritation with the term is shown by using the expression 'so-called Individualized Medicine'.

3 Individualized Medicine – A New Challenge for Ethics?

Bearing in mind such a language policy, which has to be critically deconstructed, concerning the so-called Individualized Medicine, it has to be determined whether there are actual ethical problems in this area or, if any, whether these are new regarding the questions discussed so far. When taking into account the four criteria of biomedical ethics, which are regarded as standards in most Western cultures: respect of autonomy, non-harm, doing good and justice – and adding: benefit[11] – there seem to be not only few conflicts, at least when regarding the aimed-for vision of the so-called Individualized Medicine, but the vision seems to be even ethically worthwhile; realizing it seems to be almost imperative. Categorizing something as imperative is the strongest pro-argument offered by ethics in this case.

---

[9] As an overview see H. Braun, "Vertrauen als Ressource und als Problem.", in: *Die Neue Ordnung*, 62(4)/2008, p. 252-261.

[10] The figures of the latest Eurobarometer on the attitudes of the European population on biotechnologies can be read in this way; according to the Eurobarometer, after significantly raising the level of knowledge on the matter, almost half of the representatively questioned Europeans would be willing to donate data and samples for biobanks, which are required for a stratified medicine; see G. Gaskell, S. Stares, A. Allansdottir, N. Allum, P. Castro, Y. Esmer, C. Fischler, J. Jackson, N. Kronberger, J. Hampel, N. Mejlgaard, A. Quintanilha, A. Rammer, G. Revuelta, P. Stoneman, H. Torgersen, W. Wagner, "Europeans and Biotechnology in 2010. Winds of change?"; http://ec.europa.eu/research/science-society/document_library/pdf_06/europeans-biotechnology-in-2010_en.pdf.

[11] See T. L. Beauchamp, J. F. Childress (Eds.), *Principles of Biomedical Ethics*, [6]Oxford 2009.

What speaks on behalf of such a normative advocacy of the so-called Individualized Medicine is the fact that at least all dimensions of its ideal aimed-for vision – namely determining therapies more exactly, avoiding inadequate and harmful therapies as well as recognizing and avoiding health risks which are due to nutrition or exposition – correspond to the criteria of biomedical ethics mentioned above. With that said, in the following the potential ethical fields of conflict will be examined in detail.

4 Individualized Medicine as a Danger to the Doctor-Patient-Relationship?

Such a fundamentally positive ethical reflection of the so-called Individualized Medicine is faced with several reservations. Apart from the too high expectations[12] already mentioned, scepticism is mainly aimed at the consequences for the doctor-patient-relationship: "Die individuelle [sic!] Medizin darf trotz aller Chancen und Möglichkeiten den Menschen nicht aus den Augen verlieren."[13] The individual(ized) medicine must not lose sight of the human being despite all chances and possibilities. Among other things, this could happen when the doctor, who is under the pressure of integrating more and more scientific-technical knowledge in his/her practice and is thus primarily determined by those standards, forgets that he or she should be the primary and actual partner of the patient in the fight for his/her health. In contrast to this argumentation, it has to be mentioned that the use of medical high technology, especially if improving health care lastingly, does not principally contradict to a relationship based on partnership between doctor and patient; to the contrary, it could even create space for an improved communication in this nucleus of the medical system. The circumstance that this is often not realized is a social misallocation of resources. To be precise: such a misallocation is health-politically wanted or accepted[14] – if considering the importance of the face-to-face communication for the salutogenesis of the patients as well as for the job satisfaction of those working in the health

---

12 R. Kollek, "Diskussion um Individualmedizin ist noch viel zu euphorisch.", in: *Deutsches Ärzteblatt,* 106(42)/2009, p. A-2071.

13 R. Kollek, "Diskussion um Individualmedizin", p. A-2071.

14 S. Fleßa, T. Laslo, P. Marschall, "Zielfunktionen und Allokationsentscheidungen im Krankenhaus", in: *Ethik in der Medizin,* 23/2011, p. 291-302.

system.[15] Thus, such an observation does not justify the abolition of medical research and technological progress, and it does not mean that these represent a profound intrusion into the doctor-patient-relationship. Instead, doctors have to be familiarized with the development of a new technology and educated to be able to use them, and parameters have to be created so that at the same time the talking medicine will be valued more highly.[16]

5 Does the So-Called Individualized Medicine Increase the Socio-Economical Inequities in the Health Care System?

Another apprehension is that the so-called Individualized Medicine has the potential to intensify existing socio-economical inequalities in the health care system,[17] since it would withdraw the scarce financial resources from competing projects and keep them from possibly more promising projects. Certainly, there is cause to a socio-ethical discussion due to the expectations of the pharmaceutical industry's possible profits which are related to the so-called Individualized Medicine – especially with an eye to the criterion of justice. Thus a considerate role in an ethical assessment of the so-called Individualized Medicine is taken up by the questions whether the often criticized bio-patenting will be employed in the context of this biotechnological development[18] or whether the so-called Individualized Medicine will increase the gap in health care – between the poor and the rich within developed countries and between those and the (yet) underdeveloped countries. However, it is also true that beyond all criticism of language pol-

---

[15] T. Greenhalgh, B. Hurwitz, (Eds.), *Narrative-based Medicine – sprechende Medizin: Dialog und Diskurs im klinischen Alltag*, Bern 2005.

[16] See R. F. Brown, E. Shuk, N. Leighl, P. Butow, J. Ostroff, S. Edgerson, M. Tattersall, "Enhancing Decision Making about Participation in Cancer Clinical Trials: Development of a Question Prompt List", in: Support Care Cancer, 19(8)/2011, p. 1227-1238; W. C. Torrey, R. E. Drake, "Practicing Shared Decision Making in the Outpatient Psychiatric Care of Adults with Severe Mental Illnesses: Redesigning Care for the Future", in: Community Mental Health Journal, 46/2010, p. 433-440.

[17] See R. Kollek, Gesellschaftliche Aspekte der "Individualisierten Medizin". Beitrag zum "Expertengespräch mit Diskussion des TAB-Zukunftsreports: Individualisierte Medizin und Gesundheitssystem"; http://www.hf-initiative.de/fileadmin/dokumente/ProGesundheit_9_2009.pdf.

[18] See I. Schneider (Ed.),*Das europäische Patentsystem: Wandel von Governance durch Parlamente und Zivilgesellschaft*, Frankfurt a. M./NY 2010.

icy such objections do not hold for the so-called Individualized Medicine exclusively, but they can be applied for the top health care in the developed countries in general. It has rather be stated that the aspired aim of the so-called Individualized Medicine is in convergence with the claim for eliminating the misallocations in the health care system, e.g. by not giving stratified medicine. The necessary financial efforts concerning further medical training in dealing with the new technologies, accompanied by the inquiry in how far such efforts lead to a differing distribution of means in the health care system, do not form any fundamental ethical objection to the aimed-at vision of the so-called Individualized Medicine, but they have to be accompanied in a discursive way in the course of the further development. Furthermore, it has to be examined in how far the (growing) use of a biomarker-based medicine in primary care will bring about not only the necessity of respective further training, but also the necessity of taking into account the by far more extensive time budget for informing the individual patient on the ensuing examination and its possible consequences. As said in §9 par. 2 GenDG, the required steps for informing patients regarding a biomarker-based examination are time consuming. According to §7 par. 1 and 3 GenDG, in the course of a genetic (predictive) examination and counselling, those are mandatory to be performed by a medical specialist for human genetics or a doctor that is particularly qualified in genetic examinations. Apart from the possible increase of the respective time necessary for informing the patient, it has to be considered at the same time that the handling will relatively soon become practiced if genetic tests and examinations belong to the medical daily routine – after a possibly higher need in time at the beginning of the introduction of a new method – so that only the means of expense accounting have to be moderately adapted.

6 The Myth in the Discourse on the 'Person at Genetic Risk'

Criticism against biomarker-based medicine in general and genome-based medicine in particular culminates in the thesis that the use of genome-based diagnostics would lead to the so-called 'person at genetic risk'.[19] This person could be characterized by (1) the fact that the figure of "genetic fate"

---

[19] See T. Lemke,"Von der sozialtechnokratischen zur selbstregulatorischen Prävention: Die Geburt der genetischen Risikoperson.", in: A. Hilbert, W. Rief, P. Dabrock (Eds.),

Matthias BRAUN, Jens RIED

would be dismissed on behalf of a figure of increasing calculation forced upon the individual and of increasing control over the own genetically risky body. The consequence of this would (2) mean a shift from an originally socio-economical relational prevention to a behavioral prevention depending on the individual personal responsibility, which would have to be oriented at one's own genetically risky body equipment. This would (3) leave people in a 'nether land between health and disease'.[20] By attributing more and more responsibility to the individual that is responsible for his or her genetic disposition, a lack of health is stigmatized as self-inflicted without the individual possessing the respective resources of autonomous decision making and acting. In the following it will be examined in how far these concerns and reproaches can be made plausible regarding the so-called individualized medicine.

In parts of the research of social science concerning the social implications of modern biomedicine, the so-called Individualized Medicine – besides the predictive medicine which identifies susceptibilities for diseases possibly appearing in the future – appears as a driving force in a process in which two different developments have to be differentiated at first. Hence, the medical personalization on the one hand and the social individualization on the other hand are telescoped and therefore the already existing tendency of shifting the risk from the collective ('solidarity') to the individual ('autonomy') is intensified.[21] By looking for the reasons of diseases particularly within the body and by especially looking at the individual (genetic) features in diagnosis and therapy,[22] the model which would develop is the model of a medicine adjusted to the respective person and one that fights diseases effectively – and all this contrary to the possibilities de facto given. In order to support this thesis, the "enormous gap"[23] between aspiration and reality of the biomarker-based medicine on the one hand is generally taken into account. On the other hand, it is taken into account that the promised

---

Gewichtige Gene. Adipositas zwischen Prädisposition und Eigenverantwortung, Bern 2008, p. 151-165.

[20] See T. Lemke "Von der sozialtechnokratischen zur selbstregulatorischen Prävention", p. 157.

[21] See R. Kollek, T. Lemke (Eds.), *Der medizinische Blick in die Zukunft. Gesellschaftliche Implikationen prädiktiver Gentests*, Frankfurt 2008, p. 150 f., p. 156-158.

[22] R. Kollek et al., *Der medizinische Blick in die Zukunft*, p. 151.

[23] R. Kollek et al., *Der medizinische Blick in die Zukunft*, p. 157.

individualization can only be realized by statistics built on a great number of cases and a close network of data and information – thus not in a 'personalized' way: Insofar, genetic diagnostic and pharmacogenetic interventions do precisely not break with the technology-focused and objectified ideas of body and disease as the expression *individualized* medicine suggests, but they are the extension and absorption of this developmental trend.[24] Though the so-called Individualized Medicine could presently fulfil only very few of its proclamations and promises even to some extent, one of its essential goals lies in a very different field: The guiding principle of individualized medicine does not only encourage the changes in the doctor-patient-relationship, but it also legitimizes the probing of large population groups, which would demand a much higher effort for justification without such a guiding principle.[25]

Regarding this interpretation of the so-called Individualized Medicine, it has to be pointed out that for rational reasons, the topic area of prediction should rather not be mixed too closely with that which is meant by 'individualization' in the matter under discussion here. Any form of genetic test can be described as a form of individualization though, insofar as the individual patient is diagnosed as exactly as possible. Even though the respective scientific procedures may not essentially differ in method, yet from the perspective of ethical research, law and social science it has to be stated that there are relevant differences between predictive examinations and such tests that serve the refinement of an existing diagnosis or the verification of an assumed diagnosis. The 'nether land between health and disease' mentioned above has only been entered by predictive tests, if at all. The more precise and binding the statements on the developments of possible diseases in the future are, the more do the boundaries between dis-

---

[24] "Insofern brechen gendiagnostische und pharmakogenetische Interventionen gerade nicht mit technikzentrierten und verdinglichten Vorstellungen von Körper und Krankheit, wie der Begriff einer *individualisierten* Medizin suggeriert, sondern sie sind die Verlängerung und Vertiefung dieser Entwicklungstrends.", see R. Kollek et al., *Der medizinische Blick in die Zukunft*, p. 158.

[25] "Insofern befördert das Leitbild der individualisierten Medizin nicht nur Veränderungen in der Arzt-Patienten-Beziehung, sondern wird auch zur Legitimation für die Beforschung großer Bevölkerungsgruppen, die ohne ein solches Leitbild einen sehr viel höheren Begründungsaufwand erfordern würde.", see R. Kollek et al., *Der medizinische Blick in die Zukunft*, p. 158.

ease and health blur, at least on the level of the individuals affected. Only in a small minority of pathologies it is possible to gain a relevant degree of certainty whether a disease will break out, whereas generally only susceptibilities can be determined, which admittedly predispose a certain disease – whose outbreak and course can be influenced by respective measures – to a higher level than the statistical norm. Therefore, the focus of the questions that have to be asked in the context of predictive diagnosis is altered in a significant way. Concerning this, it actually has to be discussed how given knowledge on such dispositions is to be balanced with respective behaviour appropriate to the risk or with behaviour ignoring the risk.

The initial situation of non-predictive genetic diagnostics is already different insofar as the person that is examined in a genetic or genomic way clearly already is a patient and thus, what lies in the focus of interest are not possible dispositions to diseases, which are to be treated preventively by socially building a respective regime of behavioural attributes together with negating social, epidemiological influences. At this point, genetic results additionally function as a possible refinement of treatment that has to be carried out anyway and thus cause the elimination of therapeutic risks, e.g. of the so-called "side effects". However, it does not stop with all the critical questions that can arise in the context of genetic tests prior to the so-called Individualized Medicine. Nevertheless, the necessary differentiation between predictive and non-predictive genetic tests can prevent the too rash transfer of problem constellations from one area to another and thus makes a realistic assessment of possibilities and limitations of the so-called individualized medicine possible.

To the latter point we can count the empirically obvious discrepancy between the actually feasible and the visionary possible. Concerning the view presented above, it is firstly correct that there is a certain hype particularly but not exclusively in the field of the so-called Individualized Medicine with a multi-causal aetiology that has to be observed. It is beyond debate that this hype is to a considerable degree due to the battle for the attention of the media and – even more – to the research funds which are governed by the public opinion to a certain degree and within certain boundaries. The fact that only a fraction of the announced benefit of the so-called Individualized Medicine can be realized at present is as correct as it is self-evident, if taking into account the complexity of the research subject and the methodical challenges especially pointed out by critics and not only by studies based on populations but also by studies within a smaller context.

The rightly stated difference between aspiration and reality of the so-called Individualized Medicine marks the necessity of an objectification of the debate and a realistic "vision assessment"[26], which also includes a realistic temporal horizon for achieving the aspired goals. However, there are not only hopes raised, but also fears fanned, which contribute to this hype and such an ambiguity generates the interest of the media, since the public attention may be even more attracted by exaggerated negative scenarios than by visions of the feasible and the possible. Therefore, observing the field of the so-called individualized medicine demands the triple attribution of responsibility of science and economy, politics and media, and the ELSA research to question their own contribution to the hype concerning the so-called Individualized Medicine by continual self reflexion and if necessary, it has to be corrected according to a realistic and indeed controversial debate.

To sum up: Regarding the particularly critical positions, it is important to ask whether the scenarios developed are *mandatorily* connected with the application of a biomarker-based medicine. On the factual level, the possible degree of the intrusion of non-genetic biomarker tests into the way of life, the feeling of identity or possible discriminations and stigmatizations is underestimated. Thus a positive AIDS test may have more grave consequences than a less informative genetic test on a multi-factorial disease. The latest results of genome research show that it has to be taken into account that there are intra- and extra-organic environments, behavior, nutrition and exposition that influence genes and the extent and the manifestation of genomic effects. If that is the case, the alleged risks that arise from the allegedly growing relevance of genomic knowledge not only for medicine but also for the actual way of living of the people must be put into context, meaning they have to be conceived and classified as less important than before. Consequently, it can only be spoken of the often stated specialty but not of the exceptionality of genetic knowledge. Such a specialty can only be stated regarding the social perception and the public handling of data, but not regarding the bio-scientific characteristics of data. It fol-

---

[26] See J. Grin et al., *Vision Assessment.*

lows: If the knowledge about the significantly limited importance of the genome was conveyed to the distributional channels of media, education, law, science and politics to a greater extent, the idea of being able to constantly influence one's own health by using genomic knowledge could be rejected as a travesty. It would be ethically more reasonable to respectively enlighten people instead of perpetuating such a scientifically not verified exceptionalism by using dark visions of self-imposed diseases due to genetic knowledge.

7 The Current Legal Situation

What has to be taken into account apart from decidedly ethical issues of the so-called Individualized Medicine is the legal situation. Thus the research on biomarker-based medicine does not take place in an empty space, but can rest upon established standards of human and civil rights – at least in Germany, Europe and most of the developed countries.[27] Discriminations due to genetic characteristics or disabilities are legally condemned by the UN, the European anti-discrimination policy, the German *Grundgesetz* and the law of genetic diagnostics. Admittedly, it is true that it has to be thoroughly observed if a mindset, which runs contrarily to this unanimous and decisive normative framework[28], is spreading in society under the surface and if intervention is necessary. However, the existing legal standards of protection and participation, which surely are in need of more solid strategies of implementation – such as the attempts of realization of the so-called UN convention on the rights of persons with disabilities presently show, which can be regarded as an important and at the same time stable cultural achievement, which dismisses any hasty and historically decaying dramatized vision of a regime of genetic discrimination into the realm of fantasy.

Regarding the legal regulation of the doctor-patient-relationship, the development of the so-called Individualized Medicine is continuing with the previous tasks of a doctor. According to §1 par. 2 of the code of medical ethics, it is the doctor's task to care for and recover the patients' health

---

[27] See W. H. Eberbach, "Juristische Aspekte einer individualisierten Medizin", in: *Medizinrecht,* 29/2011, p. 757-770.

[28] See C. Novas, N. Rose, "Genetic risk and the birth of the somatic individual.", in: *Economy and Society,* 29(4)/2000, p. 485-513.

and the alleviation of suffering in the case of failure. Furthermore, it is the goal of medical behaviour to contribute to the preservation of the natural essentials of life regarding the importance of health for mankind. This goal is in no way neglected by the so-called Individualized Medicine, but rather refined regarding the discovery of causes and incidences of diseases. A special focus needs be put on three aspects as definite challenges which will be important in the course of the further implementation of the so-called Individualized Medicine: Firstly, the existing consent models have to be remodelled in such a way that genomic examinations as well as the general use of collected data may only happen if the patient has generally but explicitly given his or her consent.[29] This has to be coherent with existing procedural regulations for dealing with the patients' data.[30]

An issue that will gain further attention from a legal as well as from an ethical perspective is the second question on how to deal with the continually growing liability risk of doctors. At the same time, the risk of not informing the individual patient regarding his/her respective preconditions entirely as well as the possibility of neglecting a treatment – detected as essential afterwards – due to a continually growing number of diagnostic tools or having drawn the wrong conclusions from a diagnostic instrument, increases.[31] Even though this is not a genuine problem of a medicine increasingly focusing on biomarkers, but rather a general consequence of the growing development and the differentiation of medicine; there will be a special challenge in the further shaping of the so-called Individualized Medicine.

Thirdly, the legal dealings of data privacy with the personal data accumulated by the biobanks, whose establishing and extension will form the premise for the success of the so-called Individualized Medicine, will have to be accompanied by critical-professional monitoring and the existing regulations will continually have to be questioned for their appropriateness. Here, it is a special challenge to establish an organisational infrastructure –

---

[29] See G. Boniolo, P. P. Di Fiore, S. Pece, "Trusted consent and research biobanks: towards a 'new alliance' between researchers and donors", in: *Bioethics*, 26(2)/2010, p. 1-8.

[30] Claiming the continuing obligation of the consent of the patient depending on the respective research project, this would de facto be the end of biobank research on the one hand and introduce again a genetic exceptionalism from behind on the other hand.

[31] See W. H. Eberbach, "Juristische Aspekte".

also compatible with the respective national legal standards – and above all to work at an internationally mandatory regulation on using tissue samples and data.[32]

8 Autonomy and Solidarity

It has to be closely observed in how far the *whole* human being as a person really remains the focus of the stratifying precision of therapies according to the so-called Individualized Medicine's own claims. Accordingly, the ethical assessment will be oriented towards the question whether this medical approach can contribute to reduce health inequalities in its further development. Fair and equal opportunities form the foundation of the broadly agreed-upon socio-theoretical promise of the Western doctrine of freedom. Autonomy and lived solidarity that enables to autonomy are directly linked and are mutually dependent. Where there is freedom founded in a way that all, including the weakest, are able to really participate in social communication,[33] possibly even by means of the so-called Individualized Medicine, there the call for more autonomy in the health system is not only legitimate but also necessary. This ability has to be intensively and extensively prepared and realized regarding sensitive differentiations of age, class, gender and ethnicity. If only claimed pro forma, the otherwise legitimate call for autonomy loses its ethical justification. The success of the so-called Individualized Medicine – as well as the success of the ethical assessment – will have to be measured according to the question in how far it will manage to contribute to this core of Western culture. Analogous to such a determination of autonomy and solidarity, it can be observed that from an ethical perspective a shift in the relationship between autonomy and solidarity cannot be described as particularly specific for the current developments of the so-called Individualized Medicine. Such an assessment regarding the relationship of autonomy and solidarity in the course of the current ethical assessment particularly refers to the possibilities of applications of the so-called Individualized Medicine in the field of therapy. Here the individual

---

[32] See Deutscher Ethikrat (Ed.), *Humanbiobanken für die Forschung. Stellungnahme*, Berlin 2010.

[33] See P. Dabrock (Ed.), *Befähigungsgerechtigkeit: ein Grundkonzept konkreter Ethik in fundamentaltheologischer Perspektive*, Gütersloh 2011.

patient's autonomy has always been one of the essential markers for the relationship between doctor and patient, as well as of the respective determination of the relationship between health and illness. The fact that, concerning the different questions of financing the so-called Individualized Medicine, there is indeed a shift in the relationship between autonomy and solidarity to be found; this is however not a question which is exceptionally connected to the development of a biomarker-based medicine, but a question which has to be asked in a social context: How should the (notoriously limited) means of the health care system be used and at which point? Thus it is one of the classic questions of the medical-ethical and governmental discussions, which refinements of therapeutic measures should be financed solidarily and at which point of differentiation the line is crossed and such solidary financing is no longer part of the catalogue of benefits. However, such a threshold is no statistical monument of a discourse decision once made, but rather a dynamic decision that continually questions new technologies due to their possible effect on the better treatment of the patients. In this process the biomarker-based medicine has to be examined regarding the question which of its promised applications will be realized in which context of application and which effects they will be able to show for the respective optimizing of therapy. In brief: When comparing the questions discussed with the current stage of discussion of the public health research, the so-called Individualized Medicine carries forward the classic public health questions – whereby an accompanying assessment of the further development becomes in no way obsolete, however, it can be integrated in the classical methods and questions.

9 Conclusion

The so-called Individualized Medicine does not raise completely new questions in its ethical assessment, but in the course of its further development it again focuses on questions of how we as a society want to allocate and prioritize the limited resources of the health care system, how an inclusive conception of autonomy and solidarity can be developed and successfully created and by which (training) measures the handling of new (bio-) technological developments in the medical daily routine can be made beneficial for the doctor-patient-relationship. Here the current legal regulations for dealing with the challenges of the biomarker-based medicine offer an appropriate framework that has to be (further) filled with life in its ongoing development.

Literature

G. Agamben (Ed.), *Homo sacer. Die Souveränität der Macht und das nackte Leben*, Frankfurt a. M. 2002.

N. Agar (Ed.), *Liberal Eugenics: In Defence of Human Enhancement*, Malden 2005.

R. Albritton, R. Jessop, R. Westra (Eds.), *Political Economy and Global Capitalism*, London 2007.

E. Angehrn, G. Lohmann (Eds.), *Ethik und Marx*, Königstein 1986.

V. Árnason, "Database Research: Public and Private Interests", in: *Cambridge Quarterly of Healthcare Ethics*, 20(4)/2011, p. 563-571.

Australian Law Reform Commission (Ed.), *Essentially Yours: The Protection of Human Genetic Information in Australia*, 2003, p. 33.

S. Barnoy, "Genetic testing for late-onset diseases: effect of disease controllability, test predictivity, and gender on the decision to take the test.", in: *Genetic Testing*, 11(2)/2007, p. 187-192.

M. W. Barr (Ed.), *Mental Defectives, Their History, Treatment, and Training*, Philadelphia 1904.

W. Bartens, Art. "Jedem seine Pille", in: *Süddeutsche Zeitung* 18.03.2011.

U. Barth (Ed.), *Aufgeklärter Protestantismus*, Tübingen 2004.

U. Barth, "Der ethische Individualitätsgedanke beim frühen Schleiermacher", in: G. Jerouschek, A. Sames (Eds.), *Aufklärung und Erneuerung. Beiträge zur Geschichte der Universität Halle im ersten Jahrhundert ihres Bestehens (1694-1806)*, Hanau/Halle 1994, p. 309-331.

T. L. Beauchamp, J. F. Childress, *Principles of Biomedical Ethics*, [6]Oxford 2009.

E. Beck-Gernsheim, "Gesundheit und Verantwortung im Zeitalter der Gentechnologie", in: E. Beck-Gernsheim, U. Beck (Eds.), *Riskante Freiheiten. Individualisierung in modernen Gesellschaften*, Frankfurt a.M. 1994, p. 316-335.

U. Beck, E. Beck-Gernsheim, "Individualisierung in modernen Gesellschaften – Perspektiven und Kontroversen einer subjektorientierten Soziologie", in: E. Beck-Gernsheim, U. Beck (Eds.), *Riskante Freiheiten. Individualisierung in modernen Gesellschaften*, Frankfurt a.M.1994, p. 10-39.

R. Bell, "Ongoing trials with trastuzumab in metastatic breast cancer", in: *Annals of Oncology*, 12(1)/2001, p. 69-73.

R. Berger, "'Fight or Flight?': Roland Berger Study Intensifies Diversification as One of the Most Prominent Trends in the Pharmaceutical Industry"; http://www.rolandberger.com/media/press/releases/510-press_archive2010_sc_content/Diversification_in_the_pharmaceutical_industry.html.

M. D. Bister, "Jemand kommt zu Dir und sagt bitte': Eine empirische Studie zur Gewebespende im Krankenhauskontext", in: *Österreichische Zeitschrift für Soziologie*, 34/2009, p. 72-78.

E. Black (Ed.), *War against the Weak: Eugenics and America's Campaign to Create a Master Race*, NY 2003.

H. Bolouri (Ed.), *Personal Genomics and Personalized Medicine*, London 2010.

G. Boniolo, P. P. Di Fiore, S. Pece, "Trusted consent and research biobanks: towards a 'new alliance' between researchers and donors", in: *Bioethics*, 26(2)/2010, p. 1-8.

P. Bourdieu, *Die feinen Unterschiede. Kritik der gesellschaftlichen Urteilskraft*, Frankfurt 1987.

P. Borry, M. C. Cornel, H. C. Howard, "Where are you going, where have you been: a recent history of the direct-to-consumer genetic testing market", in: *Journal of Community Genetics*, 1(3)/2010, p. 101-106.

E. P. Bottinger, "Foundations, Promises and Uncertainties of Personalized Medicine." in: *Mount Sinai Journal of Medicine*, 74/2007, p. 15-21.

A. Brand, P. Dabrock, N. Paul, P. Schröder (Eds.), *Gesundheitssicherung im Zeitalter der Genomforschung. Diskussion, Aktivitäten und Institutionalisierung von Public Health Genetics in Deutschland. Gutachten im Auftrag der Friedrich-Ebert-Stiftung*, Berlin 2004.

H. Braun, "Vertrauen als Ressource und als Problem.", in: *Die Neue Ordnung*, 62(4)/2008, p. 252-261.

A. Bredart, C. Bouleuc, S. Dolbeault, "Doctor-patient communication and satisfaction with care in oncology.", in: *Current Opinion in Oncology*, 17(4)/2005, p. 351-354.

A. L. Bredenoord, N. C. Onland-Moret, J. J. M. Van Delden, "Feedback of Individual Genetic Results to Research Participants: In favor of a Qualified Disclosure Policy", in: *Human Mutation*, 32(8)/2011, p. 861-867.

H. Breivik, N. Cherny, B. Collett, F. de Conno, M. Filbet, A. J. Foubert, R. Cohen, L. Dow, "Cancer-related pain: a pan-European survey of prevalence, treatment, and patient attitudes.", in: *Annals of Oncology*, 20(8)/2009, p. 1420-1433.

R. F. Brown, E. Shuk, N. Leighl, P. Butow, J. Ostroff, S. Edgerson, M. Tattersall, "Enhancing Decision Making about Participation in Cancer Clinical Trials: Development of a Question Prompt List", in: *Support Care Cancer*, 19(8)/2011, p. 1227-1238.

E. M. Bunnik, M. H. N. Schermer, A. Cecile, J.W. Janssens, "Personal genome testing: Test characteristics to clarify the discourse on ethical, legal and societal issues", in: *BMC Medical Ethics*, 12(11)/2011.

W. Burke, H. Burton, A. E. Hall, M. Karmali, M. J. Khoury, B. Knoppers, E. M. Meslin, F. Stanley, C. F. Wright, R. L. Zimmern, Ickworth Group, "Extending the reach of public health genomics: what should be the agenda for public health in an era of genome-based and 'personalized' medicine?", in: *Genetics in Medicine*, 12(12)/2010, p. 785-791.

A. Cambon-Thomsen, P. Ducournau, P. A. Gourraud, D. Pontille, "Biobanks for genomics and genomics for biobanks.", in: *Comparative and Functional Genomics*, 4/2003, p. 628-634.

E. A. Carlson (Ed.), *The Unfit: A History of a Bad Idea*, NY 2001.

R. Chadwick, "Can Genetic Counseling Avoid the Charge of Eugenics?", in: *Science in Context*, 11/1998, p. 471-480.

R. Chadwick, K. Berg, "Solidarity and equity. New ethical frameworks for genetic databases", in: *Nature Reviews Genetics*, 2/2011, p. 318-321.

R. Chadwick, "The Communitarian Turn. Myth or Reality?", in: *Cambridge Quarterly of Healthcare Ethics*, 20(4)/2011, p. 546-553.

A. E. Clarke, L. Mamo, J. R. Fosket, J. R. Fishman, "Biomedicalization. Technoscientific Transformations of Health, Illness, and U.S. Biomedicine", in: A. E. Clarke, L. Mamo, J. R. Fosket, J. R. Fishman, J. K. Shim (Eds.), *Biomedicalization. Technoscience, Health, and Illness in the U.S.*, Duke 2010, p. 47-87.

R. S. Cowan, "Francis Galton's Contribution to Genetics.", in: *Journal of the History of Biology*, 5/1972, p. 389-412.

P. Dabrock, *Befähigungsgerechtigkeit: ein Grundkonzept konkreter Ethik in fundamentaltheologischer Perspektive*, Gütersloh 2011.

P. Dabrock, "Die konstruierte Realität der sog. Individualisierten Medizin. Sozialethische und theologische Anmerkungen.", in: V. Schumpelick, B. Vogel (Eds.), *Medizin nach Maß. Individualisierte Medizin – Wunsch und Wirklichkeit*, Freiburg/Basel/Wien 2011, p. 239-267.

P. Dabrock, "Public Health Genetics and Social Justice", in: *Community Genetics*, 9(1)/2006, p. 34-39.

P. Dabrock, "Risikodimensionen genetischer Tests für Adipositas– sozialethische Perspektiven.", in: A. Hilbert, W. Rief, P. Dabrock (Eds.), *Gewichtige Gene. Adipositas zwischen Prädisposition und Eigenverantwortung*, Bern 2008, p. 173-198.

P. Dabrock, J. Ried, J. Taupitz (Eds.), *Trust in Biobanking. Dealing with Ethical, Legal and Social Issues in an Emerging Field of Biotechnology*, Berlin/Heidelberg 2012.

R. Damm, "Personalisierte Medizin und Patientenrechte – Medizinische Optionen und medizinrechtliche Bewertung", in: *Medizinrecht*, 29/2011, p. 7-17.

C. B. Davenport (Ed.), *Heredity in Relation to Eugenics*, NY 1911.

G. Deleuze (Ed.), *Foucault*, Frankfurt a. M. 1987.

Department of Health and Human Services (HHS) (Eds.), *Health, United States, 2007*, Washington DC 2007.

Department of Human Health and Human Services (HHS) (Eds.), *Personalized Health Care: Pioneers, Partnerships, Progress*, Washington DC 2008.

F. Dessauer (Ed.), *Philosophie der Technik*, Bonn 1927.

Deutscher Ethikrat (Ed.), *Human biobanks for research. Opinion*, Berlin 2010.

Deutscher Ethikrat (Ed.), *Humanbiobanken für die Forschung. Stellungnahme*, Berlin 2010.

J. Dierken, "Riskiertes Selbstsein. Individualität und ihre (religiösen) Deutungen", in: W. Gräb, L. Charbonnier (Eds.), *Individualität. Genese und Konzeption einer Leitkategorie humaner Selbstdeutung*, Berlin 2012, p. 329-347.

M. Dion-Labrie, M.-C. Fortin, M.-J. Hébert, H. Doucet, "The use of Personalized Medicine for patient selection for renal transplantation: Physicians' views on the clinical and ethical implications", *BMC Medical Ethics*, 11(5)/2010.

A. Donchin, D. Diniz, "Guest editors' note", in: *Bioethics*, 15(3)/2001, p. iii–v.

S. M. Dowsett, J. L. Saul, P. N. Butow, S. M. Dunn, M. J. Boyer, r. Findlow, J. Dunsmore, "Communication styles in the cancer consultation: preferences for a patient-centred approach.", in: *Psychooncology*, 9(2)/2000, p. 147-156.

K. Dörner (Ed.), *Der gute Arzt: Lehrbuch der ärztlichen Grundhaltung*, Schriftenreihe der Akademie für Integrierte Medizin, [2]Stuttgart/NY 2003.

T. Duster (Ed.), *Backdoor to Eugenics*, NY 2003.

M. Düngen, "Genetische Disposition und medizinische Behandlung"; http://www.bpb.de/themen/J6B7SV,1,0,Genetische_Disposition_und_medizinische_Behandlung.html.

M. Düwell, C. Hübenthal, M. H. Werner (Eds.), *Handbuch Ethik*, [3]Stuttgart 2011.

W. H. Eberbach, "Juristische Aspekte einer individualisierten Medizin", in: *Medizinrecht*, 29/2011, p. 757-770.

A. Edwards, J. Gray, A. Clarke, J. Dundon, G. Elwyn, C. Gaff, K. Hood, R. Iredale, S. Sivell, C. Shaw, H. Thornton, "Interventions to Improve Risk Communication in Clinical Genetics: Systematic Review", in: *Patient Education and Counseling*, 71(1)/2008, p. 4-25.

M. Ekberg, "The Old Eugenics and the New Genetics Compared.", in: *Social History of Medicine*, 20/2007, p. 581-593.

E. B. Elkin, M. C. Weinstein, E. P. Winer, K. M. Kuntz, S. J. Schnitt, J. C. Weeks, "HER-2 Testing and Trastuzumab Therapy for Metastatic Breast Cancer: A Cost-Effectiveness Analysis", in: *Journal of Clinical Oncology*, 22/2004, p. 854-863.

European Commission Research & Innovation DG (Ed.), *Biobanking and Biomolecular Resources Research Infrastructure. Final Report*, 2011.

European Commission (Ed.), *Special Eurobarometer 359. Attitudes on Data Protection and Electronic Identity in the European Union*, 2011.

European Forum for Good Clinical Practice Report (EFGCP) (Ed.), *EFGCP Annual Conference 2010. Aspects of Personalised Medicine for Society – A Challenge Yet to be Met*, Brussels 2010.

M. Evers, "Peepshow ins Ich", in: *Der Spiegel*, 23/2008, p. 154-156.

Literature

J. G. Fichte, *Das System der Sittenlehre nach den Prinzipien der Wissenschafts-lehre*. Edited by H. Verweyen [1995], Hamburg 1798.

J. G. Fichte, *Grundlage der gesamten Wissenschaftslehre als Handschrift für seine Zuhörer*. Edited by W. G. Jacobs [1997], Leipzig 1794.

W. Fierz, "Challenge of Personalized Health Care: To What Extent is Medicine Already Individualized and what are the Future Trends?", in: *Medical Science Monitor*, 10(5)/2004, p. 111-123.

S. Fleßa, T. Laslo, P. Marschall, Zielfunktionen und Allokationsentscheidungen im Krankenhaus", in: *Ethik in der Medizin*, 23/2011, p. 291-302.

M. Frank (Ed.), *Selbstbewusstsein und Selbsterkenntnis. Essays zur analytischen Philosophie der Subjektivität*, Stuttgart 1991.

M. Frank (Ed.), *Die Unhintergehbarkeit von Individualität. Reflexionen über Subjekt, Person und Individuum aus Anlaß ihrer 'postmodernen' Toterklärung*, Frankfurt a. M. 1986.

A. Franke, *Modelle von Gesundheit und Krankheit. Lehrbuch Gesundheitswissenschaften*, Bern 2010.

N. Fraser, "Von der Disziplin zur Flexibilisierung?", in: A. Honneth, M. Saar (Eds.), *Michel Foucault. Zwischenbilanz einer Rezeption*, Frankfurt a. M. 2003, p. 239-258.

M. Foucault, "Das Subjekt und die Macht", in: H. L. Dreyfus, P. Rabinow (Eds.), *Michel Foucault. Jenseits von Strukturalismus und Hermeneutik*, Frankfurt a. M. 1987, p. 243-261.

M. Foucault, *Die Geburt der Klinik. Eine Archäologie des ärztlichen Blicks*, Frankfurt a. M. 1976.

M. Foucault, *Die Ordnung der Dinge. Eine Archäologie der Humanwissenschaften*, Frankfurt a. M. 2003.

M. Foucault, *Die Sorge um sich*, Sexualität und Wahrheit 3, [10]Frankfurt a. M. 1989.

M. Foucault, *Dispositive der Macht. Über Sexualität, Wissen und Wahrheit*, Berlin 1978.

M. Foucault, "Freiheit und Selbstsorge", in: H. Becker (Ed.), Michel Foucault: *Freiheit und Selbstsorge*, Frankfurt a. M. 1985.

M. Foucault, "Technologien des Selbst", in: M. Foucault, R. Martin, L. H. Martin, W. E. Paden, K. S.Rothwell, H. Gutman, P. H. Hutton (Eds.), *Technologien des Selbst*, Frankfurt 1993, p. 24-62.

M. Foucault, *The History of Sexuality. An Introduction*, Volume 1, NY 1990.

M. Foucault, *Überwachen und Strafen. Die Geburt des Gefängnisses*, [13]Frankfurt a. M. 1993.

M. Foucault, *Wahnsinn und Gesellschaft. Eine Geschichte des Wahns im Zeitalter der Vernunft*, [10]Frankfurt a. M. 1993.

M. Gadebusch Bondio, S. Michl, "Die neue Medizin und ihre Versprechen", in: *Deutsches Ärzteblatt,* 107(21)/2010, A-1062, B-934, C-922.

F. Galton (Ed.), *Essays in Eugenics,* London 1909.

F. Galton (Ed.), *Inquiries into Human Faculty and Its Development,* London 1883.

G. Gaskell, S. Stares, A. Allansdottir, N. Allum, P. Castro, Y. Esmer, C. Fischler, J. Jackson, N. Kronberger, J. Hampel, N. Mejlgaard, A. Quintanilha, A. Rammer, G. Revuelta, P. Stoneman, H. Torgersen, W. Wagner, "Europeans and Biotechnology in 2010. Winds of change?"; http://ec.europa.eu/research/science-society/document_library/pdf_06/europeans-biotechnology-in-2010_en.pdf.

T. J. Gates, "Screening for cancer: evaluating the evidence.", in: *American Family Physician,* 63(3)/2001, p. 513-522.

C. Gavaghan (Ed.), *Defending the Genetic Supermarket: The Law and Ethics of Selecting the Next Generation,* Abingdon/NY 2007.

P. Gehring (Ed.), *Was ist Biomacht? Vom zweifelhaften Mehrwert des Lebens,* Frankfurt a. M. 2006.

B. Geissler, M. Oechsle, "Lebensplanung als Konstruktion. Widersprüchliche Anforderungen aus Arbeitsmarkt und Familie und individuelle Lösungen im biographischen Handeln junger Frauen. Ergebnisse einer empirischen Studie.", in: E. Beck-Gernsheim, U. Beck (Eds.), *Riskante Freiheiten. Individualisierung in modernen Gesellschaften,* Frankfurt a. M. 1994, p. 139-167.

Genome-based Research and Population Health. Report of an expert workshop held at the Rockefeller Foundation Study and Conference Center, Bellagio 2005.

V. Gerhardt (Ed.), *Selbstbestimmung. Das Prinzip der Individualität,* Stuttgart 2007.

L. M. Given (Ed.), *The Sage Encyclopedia of Qualitative Research Methods 2,* Thousand Oaks 2008.

J. Glad (Ed.), *Future Human Evolution: Eugenics in the Twenty-First Century,* Schuylkill Haven 2006.

W. Godolphin, "Shared decision-making", in: *Healthcare Quarterly,* 12/2009, p. 186-190.

O. Golubnitschaja (Ed.), *Predictive Diagnostics and Personalized Treatment: Dream or Reality,* New York 2009.

H. Gottweis, A. R. Petersen (Eds.), *Biobanks: Governance in Comparative Perspective,* London/New York 2008.

E. D. Green, S. M. Guyer, "Charting a Course for Genomic Medicine from Base Pairs to Bedside", in: *Nature,* 470/2011, p. 204–213.

T. Greenhalgh, B. Hurwitz, (Eds.), *Narrative-based Medicine – sprechende Medizin: Dialog und Diskurs im klinischen Alltag,* Bern 2005.

M. Grill, "Alarm und Fehlalarm", in: *Der Spiegel,* 17/2009, p. 124-135.

M. Grill, V. Hackenbroch, "Das große Versprechen", in: *Der Spiegel*, 32/2011, p. 124-128.

J. Grin, A. Grunwald (Eds.), *Vision Assessment: shaping technology in 21st century society: towards a repertoire for technology assessment*, Wissenschaftsethik und Technikfolgenbeurteilung 4, Berlin/Heidelberg 2000.

M. Gronemeyer (Ed.), *Das Leben als letzte Gelegenheit: Sicherheitsbedürfnisse und Zeitknappheit,* [2]Darmstadt 1996.

S. D. Grosse, M. J. Khoury, "What is the clinical utility of genetic testing?", in: *Genetics in Medicine*, 8(7)/2006, p. 448-450.

J. Habermas, *Der Philosophische Diskurs der Moderne*, Frankfurt a. M. 1984.

J. Habermas, "Individuierung durch Vergesellschaftung. Zu George Herbert Meads Theorie der Subjektivität", in: J. Habermas (Ed.), *Nachmetaphysisches Denken. Philosophische Aufsätze*, Frankfurt a. M. 1992, p. 187-241.

J. Habermas (Ed.), *The Future of Human Nature,* Cambridge 2003.

R. G. Hagerty, P. N. Butow, P. M. Ellis, E. A. Lobb, S. C. Pendlebury, N. Leighl, C. MacLeod, M. H. N. Tattersall, "Communicating with realism and hope: incurable cancer patients' views on the disclosure of prognosis.", in: *Journal of Clinical Oncology*, 23(6)/2005, p. 1278-1288.

H. Hahn (Ed.), *Globale Gerechtigkeit: eine philosophische Einführung*, Frankfurt a. M./NY 2009.

M. A. Hamburg, F. S. Collins, "The Path to Personalized Medicine", in: *The New England Journal of Medicine*, 363/2010, p. 301-304.

M. Hansson, "Ethics and biobanks", in: *British Journal of Cancer*, 100(1)/2009, p. 8-12.

J. Harkness, "Patient involvement: a vital principle for patient-centred health care.", in: *World Hospital and Health Services*, 41(2)/2005, p. 12-16, p. 40-43.

J. Harris (Ed.), *Enhancing Evolution: The Ethical Case for Making Better People*, Princeton 2007.

U. Hasler-Strub, "Aktuelle Therapien beim metastasierten Brustkrebs. Eine Übersicht über evidenzbasierte Optionen", in: *Schweizer Zeitschrift für Onkologie,* 5/2009, p. 20-22.

M. Häyry, R. Chadwick, V. Árnason, G. Árnason (Eds.), *The Ethics and Governance of Human Genetic Databases: European Perspectives*, Cambridge 2007.

A. Hedgecoe, "At the point at which you can do something about it, then it becomes more relevant': informed consent in the pharmacogenetic clinic.", in: *Social Science and Medicine*, 61(6)/2005, p. 1201-1210.

A. Hedgecoe, "Context, ethics and pharmacogenetics.", in: *Studies in History and Philosophy of Biological and Biomedical Sciences*, 37(3)/2006, p. 566-582.

G. W. F. Hegel, *Vorlesungen über die Philosophie der Geschichte*, Edited by H. Glockner [1949], Berlin 1848.

J. Heinrichs, K. Stock, Art. "Person", in: TRE, Vol. 26, Berlin/Boston 1996.

R. Heil, "Human Enhancement – Eine Motivsuche bei J.D. Bernal, J.B.S. Haldane und J. Huxley.", in: C. Coenen, S. Gammel, R. Heil, A. Woyke (Eds.), *Die Debatte über "Human Enhancement". Historische, philosophische und ethische Aspekte der technologischen Verbesserung des Menschen*, Bielefeld 2010, p. 41-62.

A. Heit, "Alt- und Neuprotestantismus bei Ernst Troeltsch", in: A. Heit, G. Pfleiderer (Eds.), *Protestantisches Ethos und moderne Kultur*, Zürich 2008, p. 55-78.

U. Hempel, "Personalisierte Medizin I, Keine Heilkunst mehr, sondern rationale molekulare Wissenschaft", in: *Deutsches Ärzteblatt*, 106(42)/2009, A-2068, B-1769, C-1733.

D. Henrichs (Ed.), *Selbstverhältnisse. Gedanken und Auslegungen zu den Grundlagen der klassischen deutschen Philosophie*, Stuttgart 1982, p. 57-82.

E. Herms (Ed.), *Menschsein im Werden. Studien zu Schleiermacher*, Tübingen 2003.

R. Herzog, Art. "Gemeinwohl", in: J. Ritter (Ed.), *Historisches Wörterbuch der Philosophie*, Volume 3, Basel 1974, p. 248-258.

E. Hildt (Ed.), *Autonomie in der biomedizinischen Ethik. Genetische Diagnostik und selbstbestimmte Lebensgestaltung*, Kultur der Medizin Geschichte – Theorie – Ethik 19, Frankfurt a. M. 2006.

R. Hillerbrandt (Ed.), *Technik, Ökologie, Ethik. Ein normativer Grundlagendiskurs über den Umgang mit Wissenschaft, Technik und Umwelt*, Paderborn 2006.

B. E. Hillner, T. J. Smith, "Efficacy and Cost Effectiveness of Adjuvant Chemotherapy in Women with Node-Negative Breast Cancer – A Decision-Analysis Model", in: *New England Journal of Medicine*, 324/1991, p. 160-168.

T. Hobbes, *Philosophical Rudiments concerning Government and Society [De Cive]*. Edited by W. Molesworth [1841], London 1641.

B. Hofmann: "Broadening consent – and diluting ethics?", in: *Journal of Medical Ethics*, 35/2009, p. 125-129.

S. J. Holmes (Ed.), *Studies in Evolution and Eugenics*, NY 1923.

A. Honneth, *Kritik der Macht*, Frankfurt a. M. 1985.

A. Honneth (Ed.), *Leiden an Unbestimmtheit. Eine Reaktualisierung der Hegelschen Rechtsphilosophie*, Stuttgart 2001.

A. Honneth, M. Saar (Ed.), *Michel Foucault. Zwischenbilanz einer Rezeption*, Frankfurt 2003.

J. Huxley (Ed.), *New Bottles for New Wine, Essays*, London 1957.

B. Hüsing, J. Hartig, B. Bührlen, T. Reiß, S. Gaisser (Eds.), *Individualisierte Medizin und Gesundheitssystem*, TAB-Arbeitsbericht 126, Berlin 2008.

T. Ingold, "When biology goes underground: genes and the spectre of race", in: *Genomics, Society and Policy*, 3(2)/2009, p. 23-37.

I. Jahn, M. Schmitt (Eds.), *Darwin & Co*, München 2001.

F. Jannidis, "'Individuum est ineffabile'. Zur Veränderung der Individualitätssemantik im 18. Jahrhundert und ihrer Auswirkung auf die Figurenkonzeption im Roman", in: *Aufklärung*, 9(2)/1996, p. 77-110.

H. Joensuu, P. L. Kellokumpu-Lehtinen, P. Bono, T. Alanko, V. Kataja, R. Asola, T. Utriainen, R Kokko, A. Hemminki, M. Tarkkanen, T. Turpeenniemi-Hujanen, S. Jyrkkiö, M. Flander, L. Helle, S. Ingalsuo, K. Johansson, A. S. Jääskeläinen, M. Pajunen, M. Rauhala, J. Kaleva-Kerola, T. Salminen, M. Leinonen, I. Elomaa, J. Isola, "Adjuvant Docetaxel or Vinorelbine with or without Trastuzumab for Breast Cancer", in: *New England Journal of Medicine,* 354/2006, p. 809-820.

T. Junge (Ed.), *Gouvernementalität der Wissensgesellschaft. Politik und Subjektivität unter dem Regime des Wissens*, Bielefeld 2008.

K. Kaitin, J. A. DiMasi, "Pharmaceutical Innovation in the 21st Century: New Drug Approvals in the First Decade, 2000-2009", in: *Clinical Pharmacology and Therapeutics,* 89(2)/2011, p. 183-188.

W. Kamlah, *Philosophische Anthropologie, Sprachkritische Grundlegung und Ethik*, Mannheim/Wien/Zürich 1972.

N. Kanellopoulou, "Reciprocity, trust, and public interest in research biobanking: in search of a balance.", in: C. Lenk, N. Hoppe, K. Beier, C. Wiesemann (Eds.), *Human Tissue Research: A European Perspective on the Ethical and Legal Challenges*, Oxford 2011, p. 45-53.

H. Kamps, "Deutsches Gesundheitswesen: Gut für die gesunden Kranken", in: *Deutsches Ärzteblatt*, 105(23)/2008, A-1276, B-1105, C-1081.

I. Kant, *Grundlegung zur Methaphysik der Sitten*. Edited by Tredition [2011], Riga 1785.

P. A. Kaufman, G. Broadwater, K. Lezon-Geyda, L. G. Dressler, D. Berry, P. Friedman, E. P. Winer, C. Hudis, M. J. Ellis, A. D. Seidman, L. N. Harris, "CALGB 150002: Correlation of HER2 and chromosome 17 (ch17) copy number with trastuzumab (T) efficacy in CALGB 9840, paclitaxel (P) with or without T in HER2+ and HER2- metastatic breast cancer (MBC)", in: *Journal of Clinical Oncology,* 25(18)/2007, p. 1009.

M. J. Khoury, J. Evans, W. Burke, "A reality check for personalized medicine", in: *Nature*, 464(7289)/2010, p. 680.

R. Kipke (Ed.), *Mensch und Person. Der Begriff der Person in der Bioethik und die Frage nach dem Lebenrecht aller Menschen*, Berlin 2001.

D. Klemperer, "Shared Decision Making und Patientenzentrierung – vom Paternalismus zur Partnerschaft in der Medizin. Teil 1: Modelle der Arzt-Patient-Beziehung", in: *Balint Journal*, 6/2005b, p. 71–79.

D. Klemperer, "Shared Decision Making und Patientenzentrierung – vom Paternalismus zur Partnerschaft in der Medizin. Teil 2: Risikokommunikation, Interessenkonflikte, Effekte von Patientenbeteiligung", in: *Balint Journal*, 6(4)/2005a, p. 115–123.

D. Klemperer (Ed.), *Wie Ärzte und Patienten Entscheidungen treffen. Konzepte der Arzt-Patienten-Kommunikation*, Berlin 2003.

B. Knoppers, R. Chadwick, "Human Genetic Research. Emerging Trends in Ethics.", in: *Nature Reviews Genetics*, 6/2005, p. 75-79.

R. Kollek, T. Lemke (Eds.), *Der medizinische Blick in die Zukunft. Gesellschaftliche Implikationen prädiktiver Gentests*, Frankfurt 2008.

R. Kollek, "Diskussion um Individualmedizin ist noch viel zu euphorisch.", in: *Deutsches Ärzteblatt*, 106(42)/2009, p. A 2071.

R. Kollek, "Gesellschaftliche Aspekte der 'Individualisierten Medizin'. Beitrag zum 'Expertengespräch mit Diskussion des TAB-Zukunftsreports: Individualisierte Medizin und Gesundheitssystem'"; http://www.hf-initiative.de/fileadmin/dokumente/ProGesundheit_9_2009.pdf.

R. Kollek, G. Feuerstein, M. Schmedders, J. Van Aken (Eds.), *Pharmakogenetik: Implikationen für Patienten und Gesundheitswesen. Anspruch und Wirklichkeit der 'individualisierten Therapie'*, Schriftenreihe Recht, Ethik und Ökonomie der Biotechnologie 11, Baden-Baden 2004.

H.-H. Kögler, *Die Macht des Dialogs*, Stuttgart 1992.

T. Krpić-Močilar, *Mitverantwortung für die eigene Gesundheit*, Studien zur Rechtswissenschaft 122, Hamburg 2003.

G. Kunz, "Use of a genomic Test (MammaPrint TM) in daily clinical practice to assist in risk stratification of young breast cancer patients.", in: *Gynecologic Oncology*, 283(2)/2010, p. 597-602.

K. Kupferschmidt, Art. "Falsche Gewissheit bei der Krebsfrüherkennung. Die meisten Europäer überschätzen den Nutzen von Krebsuntersuchungen. Nicht alle Befunde werden richtig gedeutet. Es folgen Angst und teilweise unnötige Operationen", in: ZEIT Online 12.08.2009.

A. M. Laberge, W. Burke, "Clinical and public health implications of emerging genetic technologies", in: *Seminars in Nephrology*, 30(2)/2010, p. 185-194.

A. M. Laberge, W. Burke, "Personalized Medicine and Genomics", in: The Hastings Center (Ed.), *From Birth to Death and Bench to Clinic: The Hastings Center Bioethics Briefing Book for Journalists, Policymakers, and Campaigns*, NY 2008, p. 133-136.

M. Langanke, K. B. Brothers, P. Erdmann, J. Weinert, J. Krfczyk-Korth, M. Dörr, W. Hoffmann, H. K. Krömer, H. Assel, "Comparing different scientific approaches to Personalized Medicine: research ethics and privacy protection", in: *Personalized Medicine,* 8(4)/2011, p. 437-444.

M. Lang-Welzenbach, C. Rödel, J. Vollmann, "Patientenverfügungen in der Radioonkologie. Eine qualitative Untersuchung zu Einstellungen von Patienten, Ärzten und Pflegepersonal.", in: *Ethik in der Medizin,* 20/2008, p. 225-241.

T. Lefteroff, C. Arnold, PricewaterhouseCoopers (Eds.), *Personalized Medicine. The Emerging Pharmacogenomics Revolution,* 2005.

C. Lehmann, U. Koch, A. Mehnert, "Die Bedeutung der Arzt-Patient-Kommunikation für die psychische Belastung und die Inanspruchnahme von Unterstützungsangeboten bei Krebspatienten. Ein Literaturüberblick über den gegenwärtigen Forschungsstand.", in: *Psychotherapie, Psychosomatik, medizinische Psychologie,* 59(7)/2009, p. 3-27.

N. B. Leighl, H. L. Shepherd, P. N. Butow, S. J. Clarke, M. McJannett, P. J. Beale, N. R. Wilcken, M. J. Moore, E. X. Chen, D. Goldstein, L. Horvath, J. J. Knoxx, M. Krzyzanowska, A. M. Oza, R. Feld, D. Hedley, W. Xu, M. H. Tattersall, "Supporting Treatment Decision Making in Advanced Cancer: A Randomized Trial of a Decision Aid for Patients With Advanced Colorectal Cancer Considering Chemotherapy", in: *Journal of Clinical Oncology,* 29(15)/2011, p. 2077-2084.

T. Lemke, "Andere Affirmationen", in: A. Honneth, M. Saar (Eds.), *Michel Foucault. Zwischenbilanz einer Rezeption,* Frankfurt a. M. 2003, p. 259-274.

T. Lemke, *Biopolitik zur Einführung,* Hamburg 2007.

T. Lemke, "Die Genetifizierung der Medizin. Dimensionen, Entwicklungsdynamiken und Folgen", in: *Widerspruch,* 29(56)/2009, p. 49-65.

T. Lemke, "Die Regierung der Risiken. Von der Eugenik zur genetischen Gouvernementalität", in: U. Bröckling, S. Krasmann, T. Lemke (Eds.), *Gouvernementalität der Gegenwart. Studien zur Ökonomisierung des Sozialen,* Frankfurt a. M. 2000, p. 227-264.

T. Lemke, *Gouvernementalität und Biopolitik,* Wiesbaden 2008.

T. Lemke, "Von der sozialtechnokratischen zur selbstregulatorischen Prävention: Die Geburt der genetischen Risikoperson.", in: A. Hilbert, W. Rief, P. Dabrock (Eds.), *Gewichtige Gene. Adipositas zwischen Prädisposition und Eigenverantwortung,* Bern 2008, p. 151-165.

L. J. Lesko, "Personalized Medicine: Elusive Dream or Imminent Reality?", in: *Clinical Pharmacology & Therapeutics,* 81(6)/2007, p. 807-816.

J. Li, A. E. G. Lenferink, Y. Deng, C. Collins, C. Qinghua, E. O. Purisima, M. D. O'Connor-McCourt, E. Wang, "Identification of high-quality cancer prognostic markers and metastasis network modules", in: *Nature Communications,* 1/2010, p. 1-8.

X. Li, R. J. Quigg, J. Zhou, W. Gu, P. Nagesh Rao, E. F. Reed, "Clinical utility of microarrays: current status, existing challenges and future outlook.", in: *Current Genomics*, 9(7)/2008, p. 466-474.

A. S. Link, R. L. McCormick (Eds.), *Progressivism*, Arlington Heights 1983.

A. Loh, D. Simon, C. Bieber, W. Eich, M. Härter M, "Patient and citizen participation in German health care – current state and future perspectives.", in: *Zeitschrift für Evidenz, Fortbildung und Qualität im Gesundheitswesen*, 101(4)/2007, p. 229-235.

N. Luhmann, "Individuum, Individualität, Individualismus", in: N. Luhmann (Ed.), *Gesellschaftsstruktur und Semantik. Studien zur Wissenssoziologie der modernen Gesellschaft Bd. 3*, Frankfurt a. M. 1993, p. 149-258.

N. Luhmann, *Soziale Systeme: Grundriss einer allgemeinen Theorie*. Edited by Suhrkamp [2006], Frankfurt a. M. 1984.

J. E. Lunshof, R. Chadwick, D. B. Vorhaus, G. M. Church, "From genetic privacy to open consent"; in: *Nature Reviews Genetics*, 9(5)/2008, p. 406-411.

J. E. Lunshof, R. Chadwick, G. M. Church, "Hippocrates revisited? Old ideals and new realities.", in: *Genomic Medicine,* 2(1-2)/2008, p. 1-3.

H. Lübbe, "Gleichheit macht frei. Warum die sogenannte Massengesellschaft Individualisierungsprozesse begünstigt", in: V. Schumpelick, B. Vogel (Eds.), *Medizin nach Maß. Individualisierte Medizin – Wunsch und Wirklichkeit*, Freiburg/Basel/Wien 2011, p. 411-438.

T. A. Manolio, R. Collins, "Enhancing the feasibility of large cohort studies.", in: *JAMA. The Journal of the American Medical Association,* 304(20)/2010, p. 2290-2291.

G. Marckmann, M. Möhrle, A. Blum, "Gesundheitliche Eigenverantwortung. Möglichkeiten und Grenzen am Beispiel des malignen Melanoms.", in: *Der Hautarzt*, 55/2004, p. 715-720.

G. Marckmann, "Präventionsmaßnahmen im Spannungsfeld zwischen individueller Autonomie und allgemeinem Wohl", in: *Ethik in der Medizin,* 22(3)/2010, p. 207-220.

G. Marstedt, S. Moebus (Eds.), *Inanspruchnahme alternativer Methoden in der Medizin,* Gesundheitsberichterstattung des Bundes, Berlin 2002.

L. Marx-Stölting (Ed.), *Pharmakogenetik und Pharmakogentests. Biologische, wissenschaftstheoretische und ethische Aspekte des Umgangs mit genetischer Variation*, Berlin 2007.

B. Marx (Ed.), *Widerfahrnis und Erkenntnis: Zur Wahrheit menschlicher Erfahrung*, Leipzig 2010.

K. Marx, "Zur Kritik der Hegelschen Rechtsphilosophie. Einleitung.", in: Institut für Marxismus-Leninismus beim ZK der SED (Ed.), *Karl Marx Friedrich Engels – Werke*, Volume 1, Berlin 1976, p. 378-391.

P. Mayring (Ed.), *Qualitative Inhaltsanalyse. Grundlagen und Techniken*, Weinheim 2007.

A. McGuire, L. Beskow, "Informed Consent in Genomics and Genetic Research", in: *Genomics and Human Genetics*, 11/2010, p. 361-381.

R. A. McKinnon, M. B. Ward, M. J. Sorich, "A critical analysis of barriers to the clinical implementation of pharmacogenomics.", in: *Journal of Therapeutics and Clinical Risk Management*, 3(5)/2007, p. 751-759.

C. Menke, "Zweierlei Übung. Zum Verhältnis sozialer Disziplinierung und ästhetischer Existenz", in: A. Honneth, M. Saar (Eds.), *Michel Foucault. Zwischenbilanz einer Rezeption*, Frankfurt a. M. 2003, p. 283-299.

A. Merkel, *Rede von Bundeskanzlerin Angela Merkel beim Zukunftskongress Gesundheitswirtschaft des Bundesgesundheitsministeriums*; http://www.bundesregierung.de/Content/DE/Rede/2010/04/2010-04-29-merkel-zukunftskongress.html.

J. M. Meyer, G. S. Ginsburg, "The path to Personalized Medicine", in: *Current Opinion in Chemical Biology*, 6(4)/2002, p. 434-438.

R. Meyer, "Krebsfrüherkennung. Häufig überschätzter Nutzen", in: *Deutsches Ärtzeblatt*, 106/2009, p. 1640.

U. A. Meyer, "Pharmacogenetics – five decades of therapeutic lessons from genetic diversity.", in: *Nature Reviews Genetics*, 5(9)/2004, p. 669-676.

S. Michiels, S. Koscielny, C. Hill, "Interpretation of microarray data in cancer.", in: *British Journal of Cancer*, 96(8)/2007, p. 1155-1158.

D. W. Miles, "When HER2 is not the Target: Advances in the Treatment of HER2-Negative Metastatic Breast Cancer", in: *Breast Cancer Research,* 11/2009, p. 208-218.

M. Moxter, "Zur Eigenart ästhetischer Erfahrung", in: E. Gräb-Schmidt und R. Preul (Eds.), *Ästhetik*, Marburger Jahrbuch Theologie XXII, Leipzig 2010, p. 53-78.

H. J. Muller (Ed.), *Out of the Night: A Biologist's View of the Future*, London 1936.

H. J. Muller, "The Dominance of Economics over Eugenics.", in: *The Scientific Monthly,* 37/1933, p. 40-47.

M. Myrtek, *Gesunde Kranke, kranke Gesunde*, Bern 1998.

A. Nakagomi, Y. Seino, Y. Endoh, Y. Kusama, H. Atarashi, K. Mizuno, "Upregulation of Monocyte Proinflammatory Cytokine Production by C-Reactive Protein is Significantly Related to Ongoing Myocardial Damage and Future Cardiac Events in Patients With Chronic Heart Failure", in: *Journal of Cardiac Failure*, 16(7)/2010, p. 562-571.

The National Commission for the Protection of Human Subjects of Biomedical and Behavioral Research, "The Belmont Report. Ethical Principles and Guidelines

for the Protection of Human Subjects of Biomedical and Behavioral Research";
http://ohsr.od.nih.gov/guidelines/belmont.html.

Nationaler Ethikrat (Ed.), *Biobanks for research. Opinion*, Berlin 2004.

J. V. Neel, W. J. Schull (Eds.), *Human Heredity*, Chicago 1954.

W. Niederlag, H. U. Lemke, O. Golubnitschaja, O. Rienhoff (Eds.), *Personalisierte Medizin*, Health Academy 14, Dresden 2010.

W. Niederlag, H. U. Lemke, O. Rienhoff, "Personalisierte Medizin und individuelle Gesundheitsversorgung. Medizin- und informationstechnische Aspekte.", in: *Bundesgesundheitsblatt*, 53(8)/2010, p. 776-782.

H. Nissenbaum, "Privacy as contextual integrity.", in: *Washington Law Review*, 79(1)/2004, p. 119-158.

C. Novas, N. Rose, "Genetic risk and the birth of the somatic individual.", in: *Economy and Society*, 29(4)/2000, p. 485-513.

H. Nowotny, G. Testa (Eds.), *Die gläsernen Gene. Die Erfindung des Individuums im molekularen Zeitalter*, Frankfurt a. M. 2009.

Nuffield Council on Bioethics (Ed.), *Medical profiling and online medicine: the ethics of 'personalised healthcare' in a consumer age*, London 2010.

Nuffield Council on Bioethics (Ed.), *Pharmacogenetics: ethical issues*, London 2003.

B. Obama, *President's Council of Advisors on Science and Technology. Priorities for Personalized Medicine*; http://www.ostp.gov/galleries/PCAST/pcast_report_v2.pdf.

A. Oberthuer, B. Hero, F. Berthold, D. Juraeva, A. Faldum, Y. Kahlert, S. Asgharzadeh, R. Seeger, P. Scaruffi, G. P. Tonini, I. Janoueix-Lerosey, O. Delattre, G. Schleiermacher, J. Vandesompele, J. Vermeulen, F. Speleman, R. Noquera, M. Piqueras, J. Bénard, A. Valent, S. Avigad, I. Yaniv, A. Weber, H. Christiansen, R. G. Grundy, K. Schardt, M. Schwab, R. Eils, P. Warnat, L. Kaderali, T. Simon, B. Decoralis, J. Theissen, F. Westermann, B. Brors, M. Fischer, "Prognostic impact of gene expression-based classification for neuroblastoma.", in: *Journal of Clinical Oncology*, 28(21)/2010, p. 3506-3515.

K. Ott, *Ipso Facto. Zur ethischen Begründung normativer Implikate wissenschaftlicher Praxis*, Frankfurt a. M. 1997.

V. Ozdemir, D. Husereau, S. Hyland, S. Samper, M. Z. Salleh, "Personalized Medicine Beyond Genomics: New Technologies, Global Health Diplomacy and Anticipatory Governance", in: *Current Pharmacogenomics and Personalized Medicine*, 7(4)/2009, p. 225-230.

S. Paik, G. Tang, S. Shak, C. Kim, J. Baker, W. Kim, M. Cronin, F. L. Baehner, D. Watson, J. Bryant, J. P. Costantino, C. E. Geyer, D. L. Wickerham, N. Wolmark, "Gene expression and benefit of chemotherapy in women with node-negative, estrogen receptor-positive breast cancer", in: *Journal of Clinical Oncology*, 24(23)/2006, p. 3726-3734.

D. K. Pal, A. W. Pong, W. K. Chung, "Genetic evaluation and counseling for epilepsy", in: *Nature Reviews Neurology*, 6(8)/2007, p. 445-453.

N. Paul, "Medizinische Prädiktion, Prävention und Gerechtigkeit: Anmerkungen zu ethischen Dimensionen eines biomedizinischen Ideals", in: *Ethik in der Medizin*, 22(3)/2010, p. 191-205.

N. W. Paul, "Die Medizin nimmt's persönlich. Möglichkeiten und Grenzen der Individualisierung von Diagnose und Therapie, Vortrag im Forum Bioethik des Deutschen Ethikrates am 24.Juni 2009"; http://www.ethikrat.org/dateien/pdf/ FB_2009-06-24_Praesentation_Paul.pdf.

M. S. Pernick, "Eugenics and Public Health in American History.", in: *American Journal of Public Health*, 87/1997, p. 1767-1772.

Personalized Medicine Coalition, "Personalized Medicine Coalition Mission and Principles"; http://www.personalizedmedicinecoalition.org/sites/default/ files/pmc_mission-principles.pdf.

Personalized Medicine Coalition, "The case for Personalized Medicine"; http://www.personalizedmedicinecoalition.org/sites/default/files/files/Case_ for_PM_3rd_edition.pdf.

K. Peterson-Iyer, "Pharmacogenomics, Ethics, and Public Policy", in: *Kennedy Institute of Ethics Journal*, 18(1)/2008, p. 35-56.

G. Pfleiderer, "Protestantische Individualitätsreligion?", in: W. Gräb; L. Charbonnier (Eds.), *Individualität. Genese und Konzeption einer Leitkategorie humaner Selbstdeutung*, Berlin 2012, p. 372-404.

M. J. Piccart-Gebhart, M. Procter, B. Leyland-Jones, A. Goldhirsch, M. Untch, I. Smith, L. Gianni, J. Baselga, R. Bell, C. Jakisch, D. Cameron, M. Dowsett, C. H. Barrios, G. Steger, C.-S. Huang, M. Andersson, M. Inbar, M. Lichinitser, I. Láng, U. Nitz, H. Iwata, C. Thomssen, C. Lohrisch, T. M. Suter, J. Rüschoff, T. Sütö, V. Greatorex, C. Ward, C. Straehle, E. McFadden, S. Dolci, R. D. Gelber, "Trastuzumab after Adjuvant Chemotherapy in HER2-Positive Breast Cancer", in: *New England Journal of Medicine*, 353/2005, p. 1659-1672.

G. Poste, "Richtiges Mittel für die richtige Person", in: *Die Presse* 14.11.2010.

R. Powers (Ed.), *Das Buch Ich #9: eine Reportage*, Frankfurt a. M. 2010.

B. Prainsack, "Die Verflüssigung der Norm – Selbstregierung und personalisierte Gesundheit", in: B. Paul, H. Schmidt-Semisch (Eds.), *Risiko Gesundheit. Über Risiken und Nebenwirkungen der Gesundheitsgesellschaft*, Wiesbaden 2010.

President's Council of Advisors on Science and Technology (PCAST) (Ed.), *Priorities for Personalized Medicine*, Washington DC 2008.

M. Quante (Ed.), *Person*, Berlin 2007.

K. S. Rajan, *Biocapital. The Constitution of Postgenomic Life*, Durham/London 2006.

K. S. Rajan, "Subjects of Speculation: Emergent Life Sciences and Market Logics in the United States and India", in: *American Anthropologist*, 107(1)/2008, p. 19-30.

R. G. Resta, "Eugenic Considerations in the Theory and Practice of Genetic Counseling.", in: *Science in Context*, 11/1998, p. 431-438.

C. Revermann, A. Sauter (Eds.), *Biobanken als Ressource der Humanmedizin. Bedeutung, Nutzen, Rahmenbedingungen,* Studien des TAB 23, Berlin 2006.

K. P. Rippe A. Bachmann, K. Faisst, W. Oggier, C. Pauli-Magnus, N. Probst-Hensch, M. Völger (Eds.), *Pharmakogenetik und Pharmakogenomik*, Bern 2004.

D. E. Roberts, "Is Race-Based Medicine Good for Us?: African American Approaches to Race, Biomedicine, and Equality.", in: *The Journal of Law, Medicine & Ethics: A Journal of the American Society of Law, Medicine & Ethics,* 36/2008, p. 537-45.

A. Rogausch, D. Prause, A. Schallenberg, J. Brockmöller, W. Himmel, "Patients' and physicians' perspectives on pharmacogenetic testing.", in: *Future Medicine*, 7(1)/2006, p. 49-59.

M. Rohr, D. Schade (Eds.), *Selbstbestimmung und Eigenverantwortung im Gesundheitswesen – Ergebnisse des Workshops zu Forschungsbedarf im Bereich Medizin und Gesundheit.* Akademie für Technikfolgenabschätzung in Baden-Württemberg, Arbeitsbericht Nr. 176, Stuttgart 2000.

N. Rose, "Race, risk and medicine in the age of 'your own personal genome'", in: *BioSocieties*, 3/2008, p. 423-439.

M. Rothhaar, A. Frewer (Eds.), *Das Gesunde, das Kranke und die Medizintechnik. Moralische Implikationen des Krankheitsbegriffs.* Geschichte und Philosophie der Medizin, Stuttgart 2012.

B. Rössler (Ed.), *The Value of Privacy*, Frankfurt a. M. 2005.

M. W. Saif, A. Choma, S. J. Salamone, E. Chu, "Pharmacokinetically guided dose adjustment of 5-fluorouracil: a rational approach to improving therapeutic outcomes", in: *Journal of the National Cancer Institute*, 101(22)/2009, p. 1543-1552.

A. Schavan, *Ideen – Innovation – Wachstum. Hightech-Strategie 2020 für Deutschland*; http://www.bmbf.de/pub/hts_2020.pdf.

D. Schäfer, A. Frewer, E. Schockenhoff, V. Wetzstein (Eds.),*Gesundheitskonzepte im Wandel. Geschichte, Ethik und Gesellschaft*, Geschichte und Philosophie der Medizin 6, Stuttgart 2008.

A. Schischkin, *Die Grundlagen der kommunistischen Moral*, Berlin 1959.

F. D. E. Schleiermacher, *Der christliche Glaube nach den Grundsätzen der*

Evangelischen Kirche im Zusammenhange dargestellt. Edited by M. Redeker [1999], [7]Berlin 1830/31.

F. D. E. Schleiermacher, *Die christliche Sitte nach den Grundsätzen der ev. Kirche im Zusammenhang dargestellt.* Edited by W. E. Müller [1999], [2]Berlin 1884.

F. D. E. Schleiermacher, *Hermeneutik und Kritik.* Edited by M. Frank [1977], Berlin 1838.

F. D. E. Schleiermacher, *Monologen nebst den Vorarbeiten.* Edited by F. M. Schiele, H. Mulert [1978], Hamburg 1800.

F. D. E. Schleiermacher, *Sämmtliche Werke. Dritte Abtheilung, Zur Philosophie 4. 2. Dialektik.* Edited by L. Jonas, Berlin 1839.

F. D. E. Schleiermacher, *Sämmtliche Werke. Dritte Abtheilung, Zur Philosophie 6. Psychologie.* Edited by L. George, Berlin 1862.

F. D. E. Schleiermacher, "Versuch einer Theorie des geselligen Betragens", in: O. Braun, J. Bauer (Eds), *Schleiermachers Werke*, Volume 2, Leipzig 1913, p. 3-31.

W. Schmiegel, C. Pox, A. Reinacher-Schick, G,. Adler, W. Fleig, U. R. Fölsch, P. Frühmorgen, U. Graeven, W. Hohenberger, A. Holstege, T. Junginger, I. Kopp, T. Kühlbacher, R. Porschen, P. Propping, J.-F. Riemann, C. Rödel, R. Sauer, T. Sauerbruch, W. Schmitt, H.-J. Schmoll, M. Zeitz, H.-K. Selbmann, "S3-Leitlinie 'Kolorektales Karzinom' Ergebnisse evidenzbasierter Konsensuskonferenzen am 6./7. Februar 2004 und am 8./9. Juni 2007 (für die Themenkomplexe IV, VI und VII) S3-Guideline 'Colorectal Cancer' 2004/2008.", in: *Zeitschrift für Gastroenterologie,* 46/2008, p. 1-73.

I. Schneider (Ed.), *Das europäische Patentsystem: Wandel von Governance durch Parlamente und Zivilgesellschaft,* Frankfurt a. M./NY 2010.

W. H. Schneider, "The Eugenics Movement in France, 1890 – 1940", in: M. B. Adams (Ed.), *The Wellborn Science, Monographs on the History and Philosophy of Biology,* Oxford/NY 1990, p. 69-109.

W. H. Schneider (Ed.), *Quality and Quantity: The Quest for Biological Regeneration in Twentieth-Century France,* Cambridge/NY 1990.

M. Schroer (Ed.), *Das Individuum der Gesellschaft. Synchrone und diachrone Theorieperspektiven,* Frankfurt a. M. 2001.

M. Sheehan, "Can Broad Consent be Informed Consent?", in: *Public Health Ethics,* 4/2011, p. 1-10.

N. Siegmund-Schultze, "Personalisierte Medizin in der Onkologie: Fortschritt oder falsches Versprechen?", in: *Deutsches Ärzteblatt,* 108(37)/2011, p. A-1904.

K. Simm, "The Concepts of Common Good and Public Interest: From Plato to Biobanking", in: *Cambridge Quarterly of Healthcare Ethics,* 20(4)/2011, p. 554-562.

G. Simmel, "Das individuelle Gesetz", in: G. Simmel (Ed.), *Das individuelle*

Gesetz. Philosophische Exkurse. Herausgegeben und eingeleitet von Michael Landmann. Neuausgabe 1987 mit einem Nachwort von Klaus Christian Köhnke, Frankfurt a. M. 1987, p. 174-230.

G. Simmel, "Der Individualismus der modernen Zeit", in: G. Simmel (Ed.), *Individualismus der modernen Zeit und andere soziologische Abhandlungen*, Frankfurt a. M. 2008, p. 346-354.

G. Simmel, "Die Großstädte und das Geistesleben", in: G. Simmel (Ed.), *Individualismus der modernen Zeit und andere soziologische Abhandlungen*, Frankfurt a. M. 2008, p. 319-333.

P. Singer (Ed.), *Writings on an Ethical Life*, NY 2000.

D. J. Slamon, G. M. Clark, S. G. Wong, W. J. Levin, A. Ullrich, W. L. McGuire, "Human Breast Cancer: Correlation of Relapse and Survival with Amplification of the HER-2/neu Oncogene", in: *Science*, 235/1987, p. 177-182.

D. J. Slamon, W. Godolphin, L. A. Jones, J. A. Holt, S. G. Wong, D. E. Keith, W. J. Levin, S. G. Stuart, J. Udove, A. Ullrich, M. F. Press, "Studies of the HER-2/neu Proto-oncogene in Human Breast and Ovarian Cancer", in: *Science*, 244/1989, p. 707-712.

D. J. Slamon, B. Leyland-Jones, S. Shak, H. Fuchs, V. Paton, A. Bajamonde, T. Fleming, W. Eiermann, J. Wolter, M. Pegram, J. Baselga, L. Norton, "Use of Chemotherapy plus a Monoclonal Antibody against HER2 for Metastatic Breast Cancer that Overexpresses HER2", in: *New England Journal of Medicine*, 344/2001, p. 783-792.

A. Smart, P. Martin, M. Parker, "Tailored Medicine: Whom will it fit? The ethics of patient and disease stratification", in: *Bioethics*, 18(4)/2004, p. 322-342.

A. Smith (Ed.), *An Inquiry into the Nature and Causes of the Wealth of Nations*, London/NY 1964.

B. W. Sockness, "Schleiermacher and the ethics of authenticity. The Monologen of 1800", in: *Journal of Religious Ethics*, 32(3)/2004, p. 477-517.

D. J. Solove (Ed.), *Understanding Privacy*, Harvard 2008.

N. L. Stepan, "Eugenics in Brazil, 1917 – 1940", in: M. B. Adams (Ed.), *The Wellborne Science, Monographs on the History and Philosophy of Biology*, Oxford/NY 1990, p. 110-152.

P. F. Strawson (Ed.), *Individuals*, London 1959.

M. E. Suarez-Almazor, "Patient-physician communication.", in: *Current Opinion in Rheumatology*, 16(2)/2004, p. 91-95.

J. Subramanian, R. Simon, "Gene expression-based prognostic signatures in lung cancer: ready for clinical use?", in: *Journal of the National Cancer Institute*, 102(7)/2010a, p. 464-474.

J. Subramanian, R. Simon, "What should physicians look for in evaluating prognostic gene-expression signatures?", in: *Nature Reviews Clinical Oncology,* 7(6)/2010b, p. 327-334.

G. E. Swan, C. N. Lessov-Schlaggar, A. W. Bergen, Y. He, R. F. Tyndale, N. L. Benowitz, "Genetic and environmental influences on the ratio of 3'hydroxycotinine to cotinine in plasma and urine", in: *Pharmacogenetics,* 19(5)/2009, p. 388-398.

C. W. Tate, A. D. Robertson, R. Zolty, S. F. Shakar, J. Lindenfeld, E. E. Wolfel, M. R. Bristow, B. D. Lowes, "Quality of life and prognosis in heart failure: results of the Beta-Blocker Evaluation of Survival Trial (BEST)", in: *Journal of Cardiac Failure,* 13(9)/2007, p. 732-737.

C. Taylor (Ed.), *Das Unbehagen an der Moderne,* Frankfurt a. M. 1995.

C. Taylor (Ed.), *Negative Freiheit? Zur Kritik des neuzeitlichen Individualismus,* Frankfurt a. M. 1992.

W. I. Thomas (Ed.), *Person und Sozialverhalten,* Soziologische Texte 26, Neuwied/Berlin 1965.

S. E. Thorne, B. D. Bultz, W. F. Baile, "Is there a cost to poor communication in cancer care?: a critical review of the literature.", in: *Psychooncology,* 14(10)/2005, p. 875-884.

W. C. Torrey, R. E. Drake, "Practicing Shared Decision Making in the Outpatient Psychiatric Care of Adults with Severe Mental Illnesses: Redesigning Care for the Future", in: *Community Mental Health Journal,* 46/2010, p. 433-440.

K. E. Trounson, "The Literature Reviewed by K. E. Trounson.", in: *Eugenics Review,* XXIII/1931, p. 236-237.

J. Vollmann, "Informed consent. A historical and medical perspective", in: A. Okasha, J. Arboleda-Flórez, N. Sartorius (Eds.), *Ethics, Culture and Psychiatry. International Perspectives,* Washington DC 2000, p. 167-188.

J. Vollmann, R. Winau, "Informed consent in human experimentation before the Nuremberg code", in: *British Medical Journal,* 313/1996, p. 1445-1447.

J. Vollmann (Ed.), *Patientenselbstbestimmung und Selbstbestimmungsfähigkeit. Beiträge zur klinischen Ethik,* Stuttgart 2008.

A. Vodermaier, C. Caspari, L. Wang, J. Koehm, N. Ditsch, M. Untch, "How and for whom are decision aids effective? Long-term psychological outcome of a randomized controlled trial in women with newly diagnosed breast cancer.", in: *Health Psychology,* 30(1)/2011, p. 12-19.

B. Waldenfels (Ed.), *Das leibliche Selbst. Vorlesungen zur Phänomenologie des Leibes,* Frankfurt a. M. 2000.

M. H. Werner, "Verantwortung", in: ders., M. Düwell, C. Hübenthal (Eds.), *Handbuch Ethik,* [2]Stuttgart 2002, p. 541-548.

B. S. Wittner, D. C. Sgroi, P. D. Ryan, T. J. Bruinsma, A. M. Glas, A. Male, S. Dahiya, K. Habin, R. Bernards, D. A. Haber, L. J. Van't Veer, S. Ramaswamy, "Analysis of the MammaPrint breast cancer assay in a predominantly postmenopausal cohort.", in: *Clinical Cancer Research*, 14(10)/2008, p. 2988-2993.

World Medical Association (WMA) (Ed.), *WMA Declaration of Helsinki – Ethical Principles for Medical Research Involving Human Subjects*, Seoul 2008.

M. Xin, D. C. Wertz, "China's Genetic Services Providers' Attitudes towards Several Ethical Issues: A Cross-Cultural Survey.", in: *Clinical Genetics*, 52/1997, p. 100-109.

A. Young, C. Topham, J. Moore, J. Turner, J. Wardle, M. Downes, V. Evans, S. Kay, "A patient preference study comparing raltitrexed ('Tomudex') and bolus or infusional 5-fluorouracil regimens in advanced colorectal cancer: influence of side-effects and administration attributes.", in: *European Journal of Cancer Care*, 8(3)/1999, p. 154-161.

T. Younis, D. Rayson, M. Sellon, C. Skedgel, "Adjuvant Chemotherapy for Breast Cancer: A Cost-Utility Analysis of FEC-D vs. FEC 100", in: *Breast Cancer Research and Treatment*, 111/2008, p. 261-267.

L. Zenderland (Ed.), *Measuring Minds: Henry Herbert Goddard and the Origins of American Intelligence Testing*, Cambridge 1998.

Web

http://www.bbmri.eu
http://www.bundestag.de/bundestag/ausschuesse17/a18/anhoerungen/Humanbiobanken/1703790.pdf
http://www.bundestag.de/bundestag/ausschuesse17/a18/anhoerungen/Humanbiobanken/1703868.pdf
http://www.krebsinformationsdienst.de/tumorarten/brustkrebs/moderne-verfahren.php
http://www.personalizedmedicinecoalition.org/about/about-personalized-medicine/personalized-medicine-101/challenges
http://www.private-gen.eu
http://www.p3g.org
http://www.roche.com/media/media_releases/med-cor-2010-11-17.html
http://www.vfa.de/personalisiert

Authors

Diana Aurenque, Department of Ethics and History of Medicine, Eberhard Karls University Tübingen. Research interests: Theoretical and philosophical fundamentals on clinical ethics and ethical questions at the beginning and end of life.

Arndt Bialobrzeski, Department of Systematic Theology II (Ethics), Friedrich-Alexander-University Erlangen-Nuremberg, Research interests: Professional-patient relationships and concepts of privacy.

Matthias Braun, Department of Systematic Theology II (Ethics), Friedrich-Alexander-University Erlangen-Nuremberg, Research interests: Ethics of psychiatry as well as public health ethics, esp. ethical aspects of the prevention of nutrition-related diseases and obesity.

Kyle B. Brothers, Center for Biomedical Ethics and Society, Vanderbilt University Nashville, Tennessee, Research interests: Ethical, social, and policy implications of genomics research and the application of genomics to clinical practice.

Peter Dabrock, Department of Systematic Theology II (Ethics), Friedrich-Alexander-University Erlangen-Nuremberg, Research interests: Social justice, ethics of health care as well as the relation of public health and genomics.

Tobias Fischer, Department of Ethics, Theory and History of Life Sciences, University of Greifswald, Research interests: Ethics of reproductive medicine and ethics of personalized medicine.

Reinhard Heil, Institute for Technology Assessment and Systems Analysis (ITAS), Karlsruhe Institute of Technology, Research interests: synthetic biology, epigenetic, human enhancement, transhumanism, social relations of science movement.

Arndt Hessling, Department of Medical Ethics and History of Medicine, University Medical Center Goettingen, Research interests: Clinical ethics and individualized medicine.

Tanja Kohnen, former researcher at the Institute for Medical Ethics and History of Medicine, Ruhr-Universität Bochum, Research interests: Clinical Ethics and theories of consent.

Martin Langanke, Faculty of Theology, University of Greifswald, Research interests: Research ethics and the theory of life sciences.

Harald Matern, Department of Systematic Theology II (Ethics), Friedrich-Alexander-University Erlangen-Nuremberg and Department of Systematic Theology, University Basel, Research interests: Protestant theology and modern philosophy of religion as well as ethics of synthetic biology.

Jens Ried, Department of Systematic Theology II (Ethics), Friedrich-Alexander-University Erlangen-Nuremberg, Research interests: Concepts of disease and illness and public health ethics, esp. ethical aspects of the prevention of nutrition-related diseases and obesity.

Konrad Ott, chair of environmental ethics and philosophy, Christian-Albrechts-University Kiel, Research interests: Sustainability, biodiversity, philosophy of medicine, Individualized Medicine, environmental ethics.

Jan Schildmann, Institute for Medical Ethics and History of Medicine, Ruhr-University Bochum, Research interests: Theoretical and methodical foundations of medical ethics, clinical ethics and research ethics.

Jochen Vollmann, Institute for Medical Ethics and History of Medicine, Ruhr-University Bochum, Research interests: Models of informed consent and capacity assessment as well as questions in the field of Personalized Medicine.